"Filled with practical information for friends and families, *When Life Becomes Precious* should prove to be a great comfort to those who feel confused and uncertain when cancer strikes someone dear to them."
—Andrew C. von Eschenbach, M.D., director, National Cancer Institute

"Like my dog-eared copy of Dr. Spock, this is a book I will return to again and again. Babcock addresses a truth in all of us and gives us the help and the hope we need."
—Margaret Harriss, St. Luke's Hospital, Baylor College of Medicine

"*When Life Becomes Precious* is written with love and wisdom and is a godsend to anyone dealing with cancer, or dealing with it as a member of the family."
—Barbara Taylor Bradford, *New York Times* bestselling author of
A Sudden Change of Heart

"When illness strikes an individual, everyone entwined in the patient's life is affected. This is a sound and wise handbook for everyone involved in these relationships—loved ones, children, employers, friends, and the patient. It teaches us how to provide sympathy, sharing support and love when it counts the most. I recommend it enthusiastically."
—John Mendelsohn, M.D., president of M. D. Anderson Cancer Center

"I am most grateful for this book. It is an umbrella in one of life's most difficult storms. Most important, *When Life Becomes Precious* is wrought of love and wisdom, and in the realm of sharing and receiving comfort, we cannot ask for more than this."
—Richard Paul Evans, author of *The Christmas Box*

"*When Life Becomes Precious* inspires hope and teaches us how to show compassion when it means the most. Elise NeeDell Babcock conveys how each of us can provide support and care to each other, and teaches doctors how to treat every patient with respect and dignity."
—Steven T. Rosen, M.D., director, Robert H. Lurie Comprehensive
Cancer Center at Northwestern University Medical School

"*When Life Becomes Precious* deserves a wide readership beyond friends and family of cancer patients—physicians, nurses, employers, and social workers should all read this book. Elise NeeDell Babcock has demonstrated great insight and skill in writing *When Life Becomes Precious*."
> —John C. Marsch, M.D., F.A.C.P., professor of medicine, Yale University School of Medicine

"Elise NeeDell Babcock blends well-reasoned research with a practical commonsense approach to living a rich life in spite of medical adversity. She adds the right dose of humor to balance serious topics with caring advice. A much-needed chart for the seas of adversity."
> —Steve Allen, Jr., associate dean, State University of New York

"This book gives you a practical blueprint for dealing with your own reactions and feelings—as well as hundreds of commonsense ideas for supporting your loved one through the long days of diagnosis and treatment."
> —Marion Morra and Eve Potts, co-authors of *Choices: The Cancer Sourcebook*

"In addition to being packed with useful information, *When Life Becomes Precious* is enjoyable and uplifting. Elise NeeDell Babcock has covered so much territory so well."
> —W. Jarrad Goodwin, Jr., M.D., F.A.C.S., director, Sylvester Comprehensive Cancer Center, University of Miami

"An indispensable guide for the people most often forgotten when cancer strikes: the spouse, caregivers, and friends of the patient."
> —Michael Korda, author of *Man to Man: Surviving Prostate Cancer*

"*When Life Becomes Precious* is a superb book. It is an outstanding resource—easy to read and well organized."
> —Gabriel N. Hortobagyi, M.D., F.A.C.P., president of the Ninth Congress on Breast Cancer

"Wonderful, wise words. *When Life Becomes Precious* provides insight into the human side of serious illness, and offers patients and families the hope and strength they need to cope well."
> —Jimmie Holland, M.D., chairman, Department of Psychiatry and Behavioral Sciences, Memorial Sloan-Kettering Cancer Center, and author of *The Human Side of Cancer*

When Life Becomes Precious

The Essential Guide for Patients,
Loved Ones, and Friends of
Those Facing Serious Illnesses

ELISE NEEDELL BABCOCK

Bantam Books

New York   Toronto   London   Sydney   Auckland

WHEN LIFE BECOMES PRECIOUS
A Bantam Book
PUBLISHING HISTORY
Bantam edition published February 1997
Bantam reissue/October 2002

Special acknowledgment to Cancer Counseling, Inc. for allowing its logo
to be reprinted on chapter openings.

Library of Congress Catalog Card Number: 96-30256

ISBN: 0-553-37869-4

Published simultaneously in the United States and Canada

Bantam Books are published by Bantam Books, a division of Random House, Inc.
Its trademark, consisting of the words "Bantam Books" and the portrayal of a roos-
ter, is Registered in U.S. Patent and Trademark Office and in other countries.
Marca Registrada. Bantam Books, 1540 Broadway, New York, New York 10036.

PRINTED IN THE UNITED STATES OF AMERICA

BVG   20 19 18 17 16 15 14 13 12 11

Dedication

With my love to Jack, Megan (Lexi) Alexandra,
Michael, Mom, and Dad

Acknowledgments

To the thousands of families coping with cancer, and their friends and co-workers, thank you for sharing your lives, your courage, and your wisdom. And I will always be grateful to you, Bob Davis, who taught us all how simple giving can be.

I am indebted to the cancer organizations and health care professionals and volunteers who contributed to my work, some of whom are listed throughout the text, but especially to: Dr. Alan Valentine, Dr. Gabriel Hortobagyi, Dr. Raphael Pollock, Mary Hughes, R.N., Anne Root, R.N., Dr. Judy Headley, Jo Ann Ward, Greg Fredo, social workers Diane Blum and Allison Stovall, Dr. Eugene Carlton, Dr. Norman Decker, Dr. Randall Dunn, Dr. James Gray, Dr. Garrett Walsh, Dr. Donna Copeland, and Dr. Charles A. LeMaistre.

And I am deeply grateful to Lucy Kim, Dr. Beth Lynn Maxwell, Larry Thompson, and Tom Pincus; my brothers Tommy and Mark.

My deepest appreciation to everyone at Bantam Books for your encouragement, advice, and enthusiasm—and especially to Nita Taublib, Jim Plumeri, Janet Biehl, Grace Kline, and my brilliant and patient editors, Brian Tart and Toni Burbank, who have made writing this book a joy.

I want to thank my agents and friends, Michael Larsen and Elizabeth Pomoda—Elizabeth for her insights and compassion, and Michael, who became my editor, my coach, my teacher, and my friend. I thank him for his vision, his commitment, his humor, and for never

Acknowledgments

accepting less than I could give. He made this book the very best that it could be.

I am, as always, deeply grateful to my parents, Barbara and Bernie NeeDell, who taught me how one dream could be turned into another. And especially to my mother, who was both the inspiration for this book and one of its most treasured editors.

Many of you read the manuscript and I thank you for your meticulous editing and your invaluable insights.

And my deepest gratitude to my husband, Jack, who has worked on this book every step of the way. You have been my editor, my manager, my partner, my best friend. You have never wavered in your love or your support, and that has made all the difference.

And to my daughter, Megan Alexandra, who continually teaches me that every day, every hour, every moment is precious.

Contents

Contents

Contents

Introduction

Kicking my office door closed, I waited, listening to my father's voice on the phone, the voice of a frightened and broken man, a sound I'd never heard before from him. Although he hadn't told me anything disturbing yet, I was terrified. Perhaps that's what happens when we go into shock. The sound of a frightened voice alerts the mind, clearing it, leaving in it only room for what is to come. Hundreds of miles away, I could hear my father calculating, regrouping, and then he spoke. "Your mother has lung cancer."

"But," I yelled, "she just told me she stopped smoking," as though that had anything to do with it. Even though I was president of a cancer agency, I was reacting as any daughter might—reaching for anything to make his words disappear.

"We need your help. We need a second opinion." He didn't tell me then, nor did I find out until years later, but the first doctor had said her cancer was inoperable. There was no hope. My father asked me for the name of a surgeon. I started my list. He wanted books. I imagined packing them. By the end of the call, I was afraid I would lose not only my mother but also my father. They were so mingled, so entwined, each thriving on the other's identity, each filling a place the other couldn't. And after nineteen years of working with cancer patients and their families, I knew his health was as much at risk as hers.

By 1993, I'd seen so many loved ones like him. I'd talked to them, counseled them, comforted them, and yet I did not know what to say to him. Cancer had now walked into *my* parents' home, the home I grew up in. It had sat on the couch, crossed its arms, announced it was staying. And although I was no stranger to this intruder, since it had entered the homes of others I loved, I found it impossible to be objective when it was sitting on my couch, in my living room.

For me, involvement with the disease started in 1974, when only families were allowed to visit cancer patients. I had to sneak into the hospital to see my teenage friend Jimmy when he was first diagnosed. After that visit, I was to see him only one more time. Together, we rode around the streets of our small New Jersey town, reminiscing, planning, scheduling the dates for a visit that Jimmy would never make, a future he would never see.

The night before he died, he told a mutual friend, "Give Elise a message, tell her I said, 'Thank you.'" I'm still not sure why he said that. I suppose he knew his words would steer me in the right direction. Jimmy knew me all too well. Two months later, I was volunteering at John Runnels Hospital, in the cancer wing.

By 1981, I'd read everything I could about counseling and cancer. I found out a lot about counseling and little about the emotional aspects of cancer. I worked in nonprofit and for-profit health care agencies. I trailed after my cousin's wife, Dr. Elaine NeeDell, a psychiatrist at Miami Medical School. For five more years, I sat in Baylor College of Medicine's weekly cancer conferences, also taught by a psychiatrist. I watched intently as these professors interviewed cancer patients and then discussed how best to help them. I met with experts, including Dr. Jimmie Holland, chief of psychiatry at Memorial Sloan-Kettering, and Dr. Carl Simonton, author of *Getting Well Again*. I went to conferences with speakers such as Elisabeth Kübler-Ross. I wrote graduate papers on the psychological impact of the disease.

In 1982, with the help of many people, I started Cancer Counseling in Houston. It was the first agency in the United States to provide free professional counseling to cancer patients and their families during any stage of the disease. Well-known psychiatrists, psychologists, and social workers quickly joined the staff. Fourteen of the original fifteen therapists are still with us today. In 1986, one of the staff members, Dr. Norman Decker, and I started the country's first groups for couples coping with cancer. During weekly ninety-minute sessions, six couples came together to talk about living and dying with cancer. These groups, which ran for as long as eighteen months, would change not only the members' lives but Norm's and mine as well.

By 1993, I was president of a cancer agency co-leading long-term groups with couples coping with cancer. Although what I learned from these couples would help me later, it was of little help the day my father called. So I did what came easy. I found resources. I helped schedule my mother's first visit to Memorial Sloan-Kettering in New York City within hours of my father's call. It was a fast-growing tumor. If it reached outside the lung, they wouldn't even treat her except to keep her comfortable. I'd seen *comfortable* many times. I wanted so much more.

Memorial Day weekend. My husband, Jack, and I found my mother in a standard blue hospital room at the end of a long sterile hallway. I lowered myself into an orange plastic chair, the kind that sticks to you in the summer. My parents squeezed themselves together on the raised metal bed, and Jack leaned against the window. That night before surgery, we protected each other with laughter and stories and NBA play-off predictions.

The next morning, I arrived shortly after six, just in time to see my father looking worse than my mother. A crisply dressed, stern-looking orderly announced himself at the door, and then sharply said to my father, "Are you ready to go now?"

As the now embarrassed orderly wheeled my mother down a long white corridor, I turned to my father and said, "Did you know you can go part of the way?" He shoved on his slippers and was off without a word. I watched as her fingers reached up from the gurney and wrapped themselves around his. When he returned, he whispered,

"That was the hardest thing I've ever done." What I wondered was whether it was the last time her outstretched hand would ever reach for his.

Downstairs, more sticky built-in couches awaited us, symmetrically arranged around a wide-open room whose large windows faced a concrete wall and a huge willow tree. There we camped out, steps away from the gift shop filled with the right cards, the perfect words, fresh flowers, and books that were supposed to bring comfort. But for those of us waiting, there was no comfort. Suddenly it occurred to me that all the books I had recommended to clients, most of which I had given to my father, didn't tell families what they needed most. I needed an objective voice, any voice but my own, one whose words would guide me, would tell me what to say to him. My father needed the stories of others who had been where he was now, people who could give him hope, show him the way. As I returned to our stake-out, empty-handed, I vowed to write that book.

We drank too much coffee, ate very little, and said even less. We took turns watching the hallway, waiting. Finally, I reached over, turning my father's wrist, searching for his watch. My dad nodded, only glancing up for the minute it took him to meet my eyes. He went back to reading and rereading the same pages of the *Times*.

Where was the nurse? Where was my mother? How would my father survive if the biopsy showed more cancer? What was taking so long?

A lanky girl with long, stringy brown hair and squinty eyes swept in. It had to be her, in that starched white uniform with a paper curled like a college degree in her left hand. Her eyes darted about, deciding where to start. There were twenty or so people now seated, waiting, reminding me of a train station scene from *Schindler's List*, except that it was this nurse who was about to announce who would live and who would die.

She quickly selected an elegant-looking woman in a bright yellow designer suit accentuated by a sparkling gold cat pin. A middle-aged handsome younger man, with a bright green jacket and polo shirt, extended his arm across her shoulder. His knuckles whitened as the nurse headed toward him. The nurse leaned in, nodding her head as she unraveled the reports and started flipping through them.

The woman began wiping tears from her eyes. Patting her back, the man guided her off the couch. They held on to each other as they left the room. Was it relief or devastation? I did not know.

Then I heard her, before I realized she was standing in front of us—Sharon, that's what her name tag said. "They have sent the tissue in for biopsy." Her detached professionalism revealed not a hint of compassion. She scrambled away.

I raced after her. "But that doesn't tell us anything," I said, anger, exhaustion, and fear creeping into my voice. "How long ago was that?" I asked. She looked down, bothered. "About an hour ago," she answered, clearly annoyed. As we had been one of Sharon's last stops, it was now three hours later. My mother, for all I knew, could have already died, or maybe she was in recovery, the surgeons having decided not to operate, not to save her, because the biopsy had shown that the cancer had spread beyond the lung.

"I need," I almost whispered to her, "to know if they have started the major surgery yet. The biopsy was the determining factor. They said it would take forty-five minutes; that was three hours ago. Please go back there and find out." I pointed to some place, some place that seemed so far away, a place I could not go. Sharon reached out, touching my arm, and with compassion filling her eyes, she looked at me. "I'll be right back."

She returned in minutes. "They have started to remove the lung," she said. Two hours later, a young bulky resident entered the room. "That's one of the team," my father said. By now, Jack had joined us. The three of us stood up. While looking exhausted, but nevertheless smiling, the resident announced, "She's in recovery. Everything went well. There's no other sign of the cancer."

In July, we were relieved when my mother ventured back to work and then to the golf course, playing six holes, walking twelve. It was a sign, wasn't it? She was returning to her old life, reclaiming her territory. I should have known better. Neither patients nor their families return to their old lives. But they do create new lives, often richer and more fulfilling.

Someday it would hit us all, what had happened. For now, we could only navigate the uncharted waters that lay ahead, waters that each of us had to master on our own.

By Christmas, I started the book I had vowed to write while in that waiting room. I called old friends, colleagues, patients, and clients. I interviewed hundreds of people, asking them what they wanted to teach others, what they themselves wanted to know, what they wished someone had told them. I began leading a support group for M. D. Anderson Cancer Center, as I was drawn back into the work I love so much.

July 1996. My mother walked into my room after a grueling flight to Houston. There she stood, silent, amazed, captivated, staring at my fifteen-month-old daughter, Megan (Lexi) Alexandra, who was doing her rendition of a dance—wiggle, clap, squat, and sway. A knowing glance passed between my mother and me, an understanding and awe at the paths we had traveled. Lexi had arrived only after many unsuccessful pregnancies, and my mother's surgical pain was finally subsiding after three very difficult years. Is life more fulfilling? Do we appreciate it more than those who have not been here? I can't tell you that. But what I can tell you is that the love I experience for my family is beyond any I experienced before 1993. And if love is what defines life, then yes, for me, life is no longer an endless trail of guaranteed time; it is a sacred path, lined with scenes like these.

When Life Becomes Precious will help you navigate the tumultuous seas of a serious illness whether you are a patient, a loved one, a coworker or health care professional.

In the hundreds of letters I've received, people speak about how this book has helped them to cope with cancer, heart disease and a multitude of other serious illnesses. One woman, a Realtor in Texas, writes, "I bought the book for a friend with cancer and read it before giving it as a gift. I realized everything you said fit us. I started using your ideas immediately. Now I find myself quoting you often and giving your book to friends and clients.

"My grandmother," she continues, "had debilitating back pain. She could barely move. I used the advice in the book and decided to get a fifth opinion. That neurosurgeon operated and saved her life. Five years later, she is independent and completely better."

Another woman, a teacher, was in a heated argument with her thirty-seven-year-old daughter, brought on by the stress in their relationship that was caused in part by her husband's diabetes. "I used the advice in your book to calm my daughter down," she said. "Later that evening she told me, 'Thank you. What you said and how you said it was wonderful!'"

It is my hope that like these women, reading this book will give you the strength and courage to talk about what matters most.

Beginning with the first chapter, you will understand how to deal with hearing bad news and recognize that you are not alone. Two chapters on health care give you proven techniques for making medical relationships work. You will learn to find the best doctors, along with how to become partners with them and make the most of your appointments. In addition, a new section on finding information on the Internet saves you hours of time. How you evaluate and research information can be crucial to the kind of care you receive. This chapter helps you know which sites to trust and teaches you how to find the most up-to-date news.

Within this book, you have the resources, ideas and stories of hundreds of professionals and families for the journey that lies ahead. They offer their voices, their compasses in the sea.

A serious illness presents tremendous challenges but also offers valuable opportunities to make each day more meaningful and each moment more precious. I hope that this book will help you find your way.

When Life Becomes Precious

Chapter 1

Eleven Common Reactions:
Understanding Your Feelings

Nathan still remembers the day he sat across from his wife's doctor. "I'll never forget his eyes, the way he stared out over his wire-rim glasses, with a much-too-sympathetic look. And then he spoke those words to her. He said them as though it were the first time he'd ever spoken them, carefully pronouncing every word, every sound: 'You have cancer.' From that moment to this, five years later, every aspect of our lives has changed."

Nathan once described the impact of his wife's cancer as an electric shock to his system. "And then," he said, "there were the days when I felt like someone dropped me down a forty-story elevator shaft and said, 'There may be a trampoline at the bottom.'

"Other times, I'd feel as if my life were a car swerving in the pounding rain, always just about to collide with the oncoming cars. Your heart stops, you readjust, not quite sure what's going to happen. Sometimes you panic. Sometimes you get angry. Other times you go numb or you start crying and you have no idea why. And at each step of the way my hopes, my dreams, my expectations would disappear as quickly as they seemed to recover. I'd grasp at anything—an article in the newspaper, a note of hope in the doctor's voice, and especially those moments when my wife would say, 'I think I'm going to survive.'"

A devastating illness thrusts you into a sea of uncertainty. You are shoved into a boat, knowing you have to survive and remain healthy while you help your loved one through an endless stream of doctors, waiting rooms, and hospital corridors.

Yet regardless of how much experience you have had with major diseases, each time you plunge into these waters is a new journey. You can never know what the seas will hold, but you can make sure your boat is sturdy and you are prepared as best you can be. And you can make the choice to turn your journey into an opportunity to contribute to someone else, to improve the quality of her life, to bring joy into her heart and peace into her turbulent and uncertain world. As a result of these contributions, you yourself will change and grow and learn lessons that you will use for the rest of your life. You will become a wiser person, a more compassionate one. And you will feel better and more self-confident about yourself, because you will have met one of life's greatest challenges. But you can't get started on this journey until you have evaluated your resources, your inner strengths, and your feelings.

The rest of this chapter explores what you may be feeling as you learn of a loved one's illness. If you understand how the news affects you, you will be better prepared to handle the challenges that lie ahead.

Couples: How You May Feel on the Front Line

It was the first session of a couples support group that I was co-leading with psychiatrist Dr. Norman Decker. Robert, a tall sturdy man, appeared keenly interested as the other group members told their stories, their heads often nodding in understanding. He peered through his tortoiseshell glasses, sometimes adjusting them in a nervous manner, until it was his turn. Unlike the other five couples in the room, he had come alone.

"Looking back," he started, "I guess we're a little farther along than the rest of the group. We've been living with Sue's cancer for two years. But I remember those first few months. I'm a doctor myself, a neurologist, so I thought the way I could help Sue was to find out whatever I could about the disease. I became obsessed. I read everything. I spent hours in the library. I spent nights on the computer, searching for information. I called my colleagues around the country. At the same time I went ninety miles an hour trying to take care of everyone's needs—Sue's, her parents', my parents', her brother's, our children's, and my patients'. Eventually I stopped sleeping. I took too many pills. I drank more than usual. I was out of control. And then Sue said, 'You're driving me crazy.'

"I know now what drove me—I felt helpless. I couldn't fix the disease. I wasn't her doctor, nor did she want me to be. What she needed from me was not to be rescued but to be supported.

"But before I could give her the kind of support she wanted, I had to accept my own limitations, understand my fears, and respect my feelings. I think that gathering information is a constructive way of coping, but when you carry it to the extreme, as I did, it's a way of running away from your feelings.

"I've learned better ways to handle my emotions since then. I talk to Sue. I've joined this group. I work out. If I'm especially irritable at the office, I close my door and spend a few minutes regrouping. I try to stand outside myself and analyze what's underneath the anxiety.

"Sue is far from finishing her treatments. We still have such a long way to go. Perhaps the rest of the way I can support her better than I did initially. She says I've changed a lot and that she couldn't do this without me—well, the new me. I think she would eventually have asked the old me to disappear for a while, for the sake of her sanity." He laughed. "You'll meet her next week. She's a pretty tough lady. I doubt I contribute as much as she gives me credit for. But I do know I feel better about myself, and that has to have an impact on her."

While she was listening to Robert, Jena's neatly manicured nails circled the edge of her empty Styrofoam coffee cup. When her turn came, she pushed her bangs up and away from her contemplative gray eyes. Resting back against the metal chair and stretching her long legs before her, she spoke about what she and her husband, Richard, had been through. "The last time we were here," she recalled, "six years ago, I was the one who had the cancer. I suppose you could say I withdrew. I lost interest in everything except the TV. I didn't want to talk. I certainly had no intention of sharing, and I really didn't care who I was hurting or how Richard was reacting. It was my disease, after all, not his."

Sitting next to her, Richard, who just found out he had cancer, continued their story. "That was a hard time for me. I felt useless. I didn't have a clue as to what I was supposed to do. I didn't know if I should leave her alone or take her in my arms. I had no idea what to say. She retreated to her corner and I to mine. It didn't take long for our home to turn into a place neither one of us wanted it to be.

"Fortunately, our kids encouraged us to see one of the counselors here. And while Jena's body was healing, the counselor taught us how to rebuild our marriage.

"This time around it's easier. I know she feels as helpless as I did, but at least we share our feelings. It breaks the isolation and brings us closer."

At this point Stephanie joined in the discussion. Two months earlier her twenty-seven-year-old husband, Mitch, had discovered he had lung cancer. Sitting beside her, Mitch barely acknowledged the other members. Occasionally he glanced toward one of them, his distaste for the meeting apparent, his look announcing, "My-wife-made-me-come-I'm-not-one-of-you."

As Stephanie explained their situation, she passed around pictures of her two little girls. "We had a perfect marriage, or so I thought. But Mitch smoked. I'm angry—angry at the cancer, at him, and at myself for not trying harder to get him to quit. I feel guilty for saying this, but I'm mad at Mitch's family too. They haven't offered to help.

They barely visit. My family hasn't been much more supportive, but then, I'm not the one with cancer. I know this is hard on our parents, but running away isn't the solution. Mitch's parents have always been distant, but I know their absence is tearing him apart." Mitch looked over at her, bowing his head so the others couldn't see his changed expression or his eyes filling with tears.

"When I realized our families weren't going to be of much help," Stephanie continued, "I called some of my neighbors. These wonderful *friends* were suddenly too busy to talk to me. Most of them are in their twenties. Mitch's cancer probably scared them. It hit too close to home.

"But I still needed to speak with someone, anyone. I called three of my childhood friends from Boston. They were there for me in ways I can't begin to explain, listening patiently to the same stories over and over, calling me just to ask, 'How are you doing?' I don't know how I would have made it without them."

Some of these couples—like Jena and Richard and Sue and Robert—pulled together when cancer invaded their lives. They came to my support group to build upon the foundations they had already erected. Couples like Stephanie and Mitch, on the other hand, joined our group because they could not withstand by themselves the pounding seas brought on by this catastrophic illness.

Few couples will go through this experience without encountering emotional turmoil. Couples in my long-term support groups discovered early on that they were dealing with much more than just a medical problem. Although the spouses did not share the physical aspects of the disease, they did share the emotional pain. That pain was as much a focus of our groups as the cancer itself.

At first, regardless of whether they were patients or spouses, the group members coped with the cancer in almost stereotypical patterns according to their sex. Whether they were responding to a diagnosis, dealing with an estranged child, or addressing death and dying issues, the women tended to talk about their feelings while the men tended to avoid them, focusing instead on the practical aspects of the illness.

These different ways of coping often led to communication gaps, misunderstandings, hostility, and frustration.

Family problems that a couple had managed reasonably well before the cancer were often exacerbated. Their ability to reconcile their differences and cope with challenges was impaired by the stress of the illness. And because cancer is a chronic disease, dealing with these problems was a never-ending battle. New problems would arise just as old ones were mastered.

As the couples talked about their situations, however, they began to appreciate each other's approaches. And as they learned the techniques in this book, they began to understand, respect, and adopt each other's ways of mastering obstacles.

Robert once recounted a story about having to wait for over an hour to see *his* doctor. First, steaming with frustration, he thought about leaving. Then he stomped around the waiting room, questioned the secretaries, got angrier by the minute, and was just about to leave when he called Sue. "After three months of listening to the women in my group talk about their feelings," he told me later, "I had become more aware of my own. When I was in the waiting room, I realized I wasn't just angry about the wait. I was afraid about some of the symptoms I was having. For the first time I didn't want to deal with my fears alone. Within minutes of talking to Sue, I felt better. I understood how expressing emotions clarifies them and relieves tension. It was the first of many times that I would use her methods for handling problems.

"And Sue has adopted some of the strategies I use to deal with stressful situations. We now understand the benefits of having different coping styles, and we are willing to try out each other's methods, thereby giving us each a greater advantage over the disease."

How You May Feel If You Are a Family Member, Friend, or Co-Worker

Some of the ways family and friends respond to the news are similar to these couples' reactions. Here, too, communication can break down very quickly, and mixed messages can lead to problems in relationships.

On Irene's first visit to my office, she brought a picture of herself and her best friend, Lydia, taken six years before. The two girls, draped in caps and gowns, were displaying their college diplomas as they laughed into the camera. "Lydia has cancer," she told me, "but I'm afraid to call her. I don't know what to say. What if I say the wrong thing?"

Shelly lived forty miles from her parents. She was just as worried about her mother when she heard that her dad had cancer: "Mom's never taken care of anything. He does everything for her. She's a dependent woman. Their relationship hasn't always been the best, but it's lasted forty years. Now I'm worried about her, even more than I am about him. How is she going to take care of him? I want to help, but I don't know how—short of moving in with them!"

Sam, an accountant for a large firm, told me about feeling helpless. "I worked with Brett for nine years. When he got cancer, I wanted to help him. Others in our office pulled away from Brett, but we had always been kind of close. However, I'm not sure how much support I should offer."

Donna felt awkward and confused even at the news of a distant acquaintance's cancer: "Susan moved next door last year. We've never said more than a few sentences to each other, but her kids play with mine. Yesterday I heard that doctors told her that her husband has cancer. I know she doesn't have family near here. I'd like to help, but I don't want to appear pushy."

Eleven Reactions

Like Jena and Richard, you and your loved ones can learn how to pull together and become closer. Like Robert, the neurologist, you can learn how to avoid becoming so obsessed that you cannot function. Even if you are like Irene and are uncomfortable about making that first call, or if you're not sure what to do, like Shelly, Sam, and

Donna, there are helpful and supportive things you can do and say upon hearing the news.

But before you can help someone else, you have to understand your own feelings. Unfortunately, your emotions will confront you before you understand them. You may feel calm for days, thinking you are accepting the news pretty well, and then you hear a song, or see a movie or even a commercial, and suddenly you burst into tears. Your emotions may change from one day to the next and as quickly as from one minute to the next.

"I was driving along and I just began crying for no apparent reason," Stephanie remarked during one session.

"At least you were alone," Robert added. "The first time that happened to me, I was in a hospital elevator—packed with *my* patients!"

Both Robert and Stephanie came to learn that these reactions are normal. You may have labeled your own thoughts or reactions as crazy, selfish, or extreme. Someone may have remarked, "You're not handling this well if your moods are that unpredictable." But there is no right way to feel about any aspect of this disease.

Given our complicated pasts—and the sudden shock that tears through us like a bomb, as well as our visions of the future—our reactions are not crazy. They are the only way we can react.

From the very beginning, you need to accept that your feelings are valid, no matter how strange, complex, or unreasonable they may seem. Accepting these reactions exactly as they are is one of the first steps in facing this disease.

"Don't judge your emotions," recommends John Stelling, chaplain and coordinator of the annual M. D. Anderson Outpatient Ministry Conference. "They are simply your natural responses to whatever happens."

If you do not respect your own feelings, they may become confusing and even destructive. If, for example, you deny you are angry at your spouse, or if you smile at her when you don't mean it, you will be sending her mixed signals. You will waste the limited emotional energy that you do have. It takes more work to pretend you're happy than it does to be honest and admit you aren't. Unless you have stopped sleeping, are severely depressed, or cannot function, your reactions are normal for anyone facing a major life crisis.

The patient's journey has now become yours. You too have heard the news. You too are going to encounter monumental changes. The patient has lost her health, her visions of the future, and her sense of control over her destiny. You have also experienced losses. You are altering *your* dreams, *your* hopes, and *your* visions of the future. Although some reactions, such as loss, last for years, others are more transient. The following are eleven ways patients and loved ones may react or feel:

1. Shock

"How can this be? He takes such good care of himself."

"How can this happen when we are expecting a baby?"

"Why now? We just retired!"

"They found it during a minor operation. She can't be sick—she felt so good."

"How can he be sick again, after all he's been through?"

"Dad just had a stroke. I can't believe Mom has cancer now."

Few people will forget exactly where they were when the towers of the World Trade Center fell; when John F. Kennedy and Martin Luther King were assassinated; or when the bomb exploded in Oklahoma City. But learning of a loved one's cancer can be more painful because it is more personal. Some people feel stunned, panicky, anxious, frozen, as though they cannot move. Just as a nation experiences shock when a national figure is assassinated or a bomb explodes, we are shocked when a loved one is diagnosed.

News of a catastrophic disease violates our beliefs about the way the world is *supposed* to work, about what is fair and right. Rabbi Roy Walter, the senior rabbi at Temple Emanu El in Houston, makes an interesting point about fairness: "We never question whether something is fair when it's good. But when something bad happens, the first thing we say is, 'This isn't fair.' "

2. Anger

> "I'm furious at the cancer for entering our lives."
>
> "My husband and I have been fighting about our finances for two years. Now he has cancer. Yet I can't just forget how he acted before, how inconsiderate, nasty, and rigid he was. I'm still furious."
>
> "I'm mad because my in-laws want to visit only when it's convenient for them."
>
> "I'm angry at the doctor for taking so long to find the cancer."
>
> "I hate waiting. Can't these doctors figure out how to schedule patients?"
>
> "I'm angry that she isn't doing more to take care of herself."

If you were angry at your loved one before the diagnosis was made, the cause of that anger may seem trivial now. But if the cause is a series of complex issues, the anger probably won't disappear. You will still have to resolve it, if possible.

Anger is sometimes hard to identify. You may have the type of anger that Chaplain Steve Thorney, from the Texas Medical Center, refers to as "airball anger." It's anger that you cannot understand, and it's just as real as anger that may make sense to you. When cancer blasts your life apart, it's normal to get angry.

Many of us are brought up to believe that anger is bad. Others are taught "not that the feeling is bad but [that] the behavior accompanying it is often unacceptable," explains nurse Mary Hughes, who has served on the board of directors of Houston's American Cancer Society division.

Yet, acknowledging anger is good and has positive benefits. Once you know you are angry, you can use it as fuel to solve problems, to become assertive, and to get your needs met.

Ignoring your anger, however, is bad. It's like burying a volcano and hoping it won't explode.

3. Fear

> "I'm afraid of getting too close or being too pushy."
> "I'm scared about the way Mama is handling the disease."
> "I'm afraid of how this will affect my children."
> "I'm scared to ask for help."
> "I'm afraid this will kill her no matter how good the prognosis."
> "I'm afraid I won't be able to handle the pain."

Even when the patient has a good prognosis, you may worry about her survival. In one of my couples groups, all the patients had been told that their disease had a high cure rate. Yet the first topic the couples wanted to discuss was dying. One woman summed up their feelings: "When my husband's life was threatened, I was faced not only with his mortality but with my own as well."

Modern medicine has achieved exceptional cure rates, and more than nine million cancer survivors are alive today. But those numbers can be meaningless if your loved one's life is threatened.

Your fears may be either concrete or abstract. They may seem minor or monumental. You may be afraid of your new responsibilities, of inadequate insurance coverage, or of being abandoned if the patient dies. You may fear the experts, the tests, or your own ability to help the patient through the side effects of treatment.

It is natural to be afraid of the unknown. The only thing that is known for certain is that a complex catastrophic illness has just hit and no one can predict the outcome. A crisis of this magnitude would spark fear in almost everyone.

4. Burdens Are Insurmountable

> "If someone asks me to do one more thing, I feel like I could kill him."
>
> "I'm losing my patience with everyone—there's just too much to handle."

More than likely, numerous responsibilities have instantly been added to your already busy life. At first you tackle them by charging ahead, taking on all of your new chores as well as your old ones. You try to handle each and every one of them yourself. At some point, and probably very quickly, you feel exhausted and overwhelmed. You cannot handle them all yourself, nor should you expect to be able to. Such expectations will inevitably go unfulfilled, and berating or blaming yourself will lessen your ability to meet any of your responsibilities.

5. Loss of Control

> "I feel so helpless, so powerless against the disease."
>
> "It's not even in my body. I wish I had it instead of my wife."
>
> "The doctors have all the power. I feel helpless and naive in dealing with them."
>
> "I used to be able to manage my career, my family, and my household. When my wife got cancer, I felt like I couldn't manage any of them."

Family members and other loved ones have an especially difficult time dealing with the illness because they are on the outside looking in. They cannot fix it. They cannot see it. Not knowing what is going on and always having to rely on others for information can leave them feeling powerless.

6. Grief

> "I grieve for what we've lost and what we're going to lose."
>
> "I'm grieving the loss not only of his health but of everything it meant to our marriage. The long, relaxing weekends playing golf are gone forever."
>
> "I find myself crying when I see people walking together or holding hands or laughing. I suppose I'm grieving those times when our lives appeared as carefree."

From the moment this disease storms in and turns your world upside down, you experience losses. You experience some losses right away and others later on, as the illness progresses. Dreams, finances, roles, and relationships as you have known them are destroyed or, at the very least, altered forever.

Grief is the natural way to respond to loss. Suppressing or denying grief is not only abnormal, it will have a detrimental effect on your well-being. Suppressed grief can be extremely volatile.

7. Guilt

> "What was I thinking when I yelled at her? How could I have been so unfair?"
>
> "Sometimes I wish she'd go quickly and peacefully. Then I feel guilty for wishing that."
>
> "I know I should call more, but I can't handle having to go through my stepfather to reach my mother."

Guilt occurs when, in retrospect, you think you should have done something differently, or should not have done it at all. You *should* have pushed your husband to get to the doctor sooner. You *shouldn't* be spending so much time with an ill parent because you are neglecting your children. You *should* be doing everything better. You *shouldn't* resent people who are healthy.

You feel guilty when you do not meet your own expectations. You expect yourself to be perfect in a role that has no written job description, a role that is unpredictable from day to day, a role that depletes every bit of your energy.

If the patient is a friend, co-worker, or neighbor, you may feel guilty that you haven't called more often, or provided enough support, or made time to visit, or that you said something you later regretted.

Guilt is a vicious cycle. Once you allow yourself to feel guilty, you can go in circles, never feeling that you've done enough to make up for whatever you think you did wrong.

8. Anxiety

> "What's the doctor going to say when she emerges
> from the operating room?"
> "What are the test results going to show?"
> "What will happen to me, to our house, to our
> children?"

You may find yourself getting tense, worried, and short-tempered more often than before. You may be sleeping less, forgetting things, or making poor decisions. Your anxiety can come and go unexpectedly. Like some forms of anger and guilt, its origins may elude you. Anxiety can emerge from seemingly unrelated circumstances or from fear of the unknown. If you knew what was going to happen, you might not feel anxious.

9. A Reevaluation of Beliefs

> "I always thought I could turn to my faith, but I'm not
> sure what that means anymore."
> "I'm angry at God, but I was taught such feelings are
> bad."

"I feel closer to God than I've ever felt."

"I believed God would give me strength, and now I
have none."

"How could God let this happen?"

Living with a serious illness can affect your spiritual beliefs. It may make them stronger or weaker, or you may develop an entirely new interpretation of what is sacred. Many people use this experience as an opportunity to strengthen their spirituality. Others lose their faith altogether.

This is the time to reevaluate your beliefs. It may be the hardest work you've ever done, but it can also be the most rewarding.

10. The Desire to Bargain

"If You let her survive the surgery, I'll be a better son."

"If You don't let him suffer, I won't get mad when he's
mean."

"Please, God, let them only find the cancer in one place.
If they do, I'll..."

"If You make this scan turn out okay, I will appreciate
him more."

You may find yourself bargaining or negotiating with Whomever you pray to, hoping that by making a promise you will improve the situation. When my mother was diagnosed with lung cancer, I found myself outside her operating room, negotiating, "If You let her live, I'll..." Bargaining gives us a sense that we can do something. We can play a role. We can help.

11. Hope

"I hope he won't suffer like my pa did."

"I hope she will beat this."

"I hope we are preparing our children well enough for
what may happen."

"I hope our experience can help and teach others."
"I hope I can learn lessons from this, such as how to be more considerate and compassionate."

As soon as I heard that my mother had cancer, I looked for reasons to hope. As long as we could get her to the right doctors, I believed she would make it, she would survive.

And it can be amazing what you hope for. If my mother awoke from surgery with two lungs, it would mean there was nothing the doctors could do to help her. Until the morning of her surgery, I could not imagine ever hoping my mother would have one lung.

Last year, we hoped that my parents could spend Christmas with my eight-month-old daughter. This year, we are still hoping that the cancer will not return and that we can find a specialist to reduce the chronic pain she now experiences as a result of the surgery.

When my grandfather was diagnosed with bladder cancer in October, I hoped that he wouldn't have side effects from the treatment. When my grandmother died shortly before Christmas, I hoped I would be able to provide the emotional support he needed.

By March, I hoped the doctors would proclaim he was cancer free. Once they did, I started to hope that the videos of his great-granddaughter, which I sent regularly, would bring him joy. In the midst of even your darkest days, you may discover you have many hopes.

Turning Your Reactions into Positive Changes

Patients and their loved ones often say things like, "I wish it hadn't taken a catastrophic illness for me to appreciate my life." Because much of this disease was beyond their control, they learned to focus on what they could control.

Thousands of cancer patients and their loved ones have reported that their relationships became stronger after the diagnosis and that their communication with others improved. They valued their families more. They took better care of themselves.

Of the many families who participated in Cancer Counseling's individual, family, and group therapy sessions, 80 percent reported an improvement in their children's grades. More than 90 percent said their family relationships were closer. And some family members spoke to each other for the first time in years.

When I first met Keith, the forty-year-old son of a patient, he was perched on top of a file cabinet in a corner of my very cramped office. It was as far away as he could get from his father, who was sitting on a couch between Keith's sister and mother. Keith would not look his father in the eye. The tension between them permeated the room. When I asked Keith why he had even come to the meeting, he pointed toward his mother and said, "For her."

Three months later, I came across Keith in the hall, his arm around his father. They were on their way to the weekly dinner that followed their counseling session. I asked how he was doing. Grinning, Keith replied, "I don't know what I was thinking when I stopped talking to him. I love this man." Squeezing his father's shoulders, he added, "If it weren't for the cancer, my dad and I would have continued to avoid each other, as we had for almost fourteen years."

STRESS-REDUCING TECHNIQUES

It's hard to believe that a devastating illness—and the range of emotions it produces—can lead to positive changes in your life. But neither the disease nor these emotions by themselves will alter your life; it's how you face and address them that will.

Practice the techniques that follow and you will discover simple yet powerful strategies for uncovering the gifts within any disease. These gifts come in many forms: strengthened relationships, new perspectives, and deepened faith. You have been summoned to meet a monumental challenge. With these techniques you'll use that challenge to change your life.

Take time out.

Taking time out for yourself is a way of getting your bearings. A fifteen-minute walk is one way to do it. If you cannot go outdoors, go to another part of your building and walk through the hallways. If you don't want to walk, then sit quietly in your office with the door closed and your phone turned off. One woman used to take extra-long showers at night. It was the only place where she could have privacy.

If you can, exercise three times a week for thirty minutes at a time. It will give you an opportunity to contemplate your thoughts while easing some of the stress.

Keep a journal.

A journal is a tool to record your life and to reflect upon it later. Sometimes just writing about your feelings enables you to be more objective. As Bill Martin, author of *My Prostate and Me,* says, "Loved ones and patients can put the cancer experience on paper and gain some distance from it." Keeping a journal also forces you to spend time alone, and reading it months later can show you what progress you have made.

Start by taking twenty minutes every day to write down your feelings. During your "time out" write down what your emotions are at that moment. Then list five things you are thankful for that happened that day. List three things you learned and/or three challenges you overcame.

Writing can be a way of organizing your thoughts, a way to let go, and a vehicle to release your emotions. One nurse wrote in her journal every night in order to defuse her often intense emotions. Breaking the tips of pencils, she would lash out at the paper. Often she wrote letters to people she was angry at, tearing out the pages when she was done. It was a safe place to discharge her feelings on a daily basis. She always felt better afterward.

Reach out for support.

Another way to help yourself is to share your life with people who care about you. One nurse told me, "The support of my friends always fortifies me. They help me keep my life in perspective. They give me the strength to take care of myself, my patients, and my family."

Call a friend or family member. The friend may be one you haven't talked to in months, or a childhood confidante—the kind you can talk to only once a year yet immediately pick up where you left off. Make sure it's someone who does not judge you, someone who simply listens well.

Celebrate the smaller victories and events.

Celebrate the milestones, events, and victories that you previously took for granted. Celebrate each step you take and each challenge you had the courage to meet. Take pride in and be grateful for the lessons you learn, the skills you develop, and the new perspectives you acquire.

Pay more attention to life's precious gifts that you may once have ignored: to children laughing, your loved one smiling, a full moon towering over the trees, or the smell of your favorite flowers.

If you adopt only one of all the techniques in this section, this one will be the most valuable. As you begin to better appreciate your surroundings and the events in your life, you will feel more fulfilled, more hopeful, and more grateful for what you do have. This is a way to take care of yourself that I learned not only from health care professionals but from patients and their loved ones. They made life meaningful by embracing every aspect of it, by noticing everything around them, and by taking joy in things that others may never notice.

Learn to laugh.

In one family I worked with, a child whose father had cancer started to laugh during a session. The other family members criticized him for laughing. His mother said, "How can you laugh when your father is so ill?" But laughter is physically and emotionally rejuvenating. It cleanses the mind as well as the body, and it raises the level of endorphins, the body's natural healing mechanism.

Health care workers use laughter to break tension. In hospital rooms and in support groups, humor is often the best way to break down the isolation and bring people closer.

Don't laugh *at* a patient. Instead, laugh at the ironies, the problems, the ridiculous things that happen. Laughter will help you and your loved one put tragedy into perspective. Laughter is chicken soup for the soul.

By taking time out, you allow yourself to acknowledge what has happened and to adjust to it. Writing helps you put distance between you and your thoughts. By talking with others, you can share the changes in your life. Celebration, contemplation, and laughter make life more precious.

These five techniques can help you gain a new perspective. You will reduce some of the tension and discover joy during times you would least expect to. More important, you will increase your ability to support your loved one, which will in itself make you feel good. Finally, these techniques will help you attend to your own needs. (Chapter 6 offers still more ways for you to take care of yourself.)

The next chapter explores the barriers that may be preventing you from reaching out and supporting your loved one. Have you neglected to call someone who you know is hurting? Are you withholding your feelings rather than openly sharing them? Are you telling the person about some of your feelings but keeping others to yourself? Are you telling one parent everything, while saying little to the other in order to protect him?

You can learn to identify, evaluate, and overcome the obstacles to giving support, obstacles and fears that can be so debilitating that you don't even speak about what matters most. Understanding your fears gives you the knowledge and control necessary to overcome them. You will then be empowered to reach out and support the person who needs you. Such understanding is a sturdy boat that can carry both of you through the dangerous waters that lie ahead.

Chapter 2

Why We Stop Talking When
We Need to Start:
How Our Fears Divide Us

"Silent presence is always better than silent absence."
—Chaplain Steve Thorney

We don't always reach out the minute a friend is diagnosed. We make excuses. Days go by. Weeks. We are so uncomfortable making that first contact that sometimes we never do pick up the phone to call. We mean to. We care so much. We just can't.

There are times when many of us are afraid to give our friends the support they need. A therapist who was leading a family support group confessed to me, "I have a friend who has cancer. I know she needs me, but I haven't contacted her. I'm not sure why I haven't called, and it bothers me a lot. What is wrong with me?" He was a very caring, compassionate man, but in this instance, his fears were preventing him from reaching out. We talked for a while as he sorted through his feelings. Once he finally expressed them, he was able to contact his friend. You too can learn to understand and express your feelings and to reach out as he did.

If the person with cancer is someone you live with, an entirely different set of fears may arise. Your fears may keep you from talking about the most important aspect of the disease—how it affects you, how it changes everything you believed in, trusted in, and depended upon. Until you can understand and express these fears, you cannot fully and unconditionally support someone else.

But why can't we talk about it? For years, we have been taught that the word *cancer* is synonymous with death, sadness, and pain. In 1982, when I started Cancer Counseling, people criticized me. "Change the name," they said. "Take out the word *cancer*. Make it more upbeat, less obvious. Don't you understand? People don't *want* to talk about cancer."

Although a lot has changed since 1982, your loved one's life is now threatened by the disease. Even when the prognosis is good, your fear of losing that person will still be ever present. Of all the reactions people have to a loved one's illness, fear is the most common.

Supporting someone who is facing a catastrophic illness is an enormous job—a job so demanding that it presents monumental problems from the very beginning. But it can also be a time of growth, a time when you learn about relationships, develop new skills, and come to appreciate life as you never have before. Most important, it can be a time when you grow closer to your loved one.

No one wants to learn about life this way. And yet, if you discover the good within this tragedy, if you grow from it, if you help the person you care about, your life will change dramatically. You may not be able to change the outcome of the illness, but you can make your life and theirs even more precious than it was before the cancer.

As you read this chapter, you may feel regret at ways you have acted toward your friend or loved one. Everyone makes mistakes and will continue to make them. Let it go. What matters most is your compassion, your honesty, and your presence. What matters is that you are making an effort to give of yourself.

The first part of this chapter is for the friends, relatives, and co-workers of the person who is ill and her family. The next section is for the family and loved ones—those living with him or her, the primary caregivers.

What's Stopping You?

There are many reasons why you may not want to talk to someone who has been touched by a catastrophic illness. Do any of the following possibilities fit your situation?

"I'm afraid because I'm not ready to talk about cancer."

One of the greatest gifts you have to offer someone in pain is your presence. All you need to do is sit with him and listen to him, without saying much or giving advice. Simply by listening you let him know you care. You don't need to be prepared to talk about the illness yourself, but you do need to be able to listen to him talk about it if he wants to. If your friend has a lot of questions, you can always say, "I don't know much about this, but I can find someone who does."

"I'm afraid of saying the wrong thing."

You care so much that you are afraid that if you say or do the wrong thing, you will hurt your friend. But simple statements of love and concern are all you need to convey.

> "I'm sorry."
> "I'm so sorry to learn you are ill. I love you, and I want to be available to you and your family."
> "I don't know what to say, but I was worried and wanted to see how you are."

"I'm calling because I'm concerned, and I need to see
how you are. Would it help if you talked about it? I
haven't been through this myself, but I can listen."

More suggestions on what to say to your loved one or friend are
given in Chapters 3 and 4.

"I'm afraid to disturb him before the surgery. I will call afterward."

Janet and Steve joined my couples group two years after doctors
had discovered her cancer. "At first, we only heard from a few
friends," Steve remembers. "We quickly discovered how some people
act when they are needed most."

Two weeks after the initial diagnosis was made, Janet had surgery.
"The days and nights leading up to the operation were the worst I've
ever been through," she explains. "I've never felt so alone. To this day
the experience has affected some of my relationships.

"I also have trouble trusting the people who didn't call for months.
And how can I trust the friends who didn't show up until they knew
I was in remission? Will they disappear again if it comes back?"

Janet was fortunate—she survived the surgery. In time, she and
Steve realized most of their friends actually did care a great deal but
had been afraid to contact them. "But what if she hadn't made it?"
Steve wonders. "Those people who waited to call would have missed
their opportunity to let her know how much they loved her."

Your friend may have a great prognosis. The treatment may not
even include surgery. But she and her family are smack in the middle
of a huge battle, and at the very least her hopes and dreams have been
shattered. She needs you now. Janet concludes, "It was like facing my
worst nightmare—and having the added burden of thinking, 'My
friends don't even care.' "

"If I mention her illness, I'll depress her."

"People said I was upbeat all the time," says Eugene, a very outgoing
forty-one-year-old patient. "I was always kidding and had a positive

attitude. So most people didn't call me when they first found out I had cancer. Those who did call, didn't bring it up. I kept right on joking and kidding as though nothing had happened, because I sensed it was what they expected of me."

Eugene had just completed three years of chemotherapy when he joined one of my support groups. He was upset that his friends wouldn't talk about the cancer. Even when *he* brought it up, they changed the subject.

"I appreciate the few people who do encourage me to share all my feelings," he says. "They validate my emotions. Talking about painful topics doesn't depress me—it helps me to keep my sanity."

"I'm afraid we won't have anything to say to each other. We've never talked about cancer before."

You have a relationship with this person. Don't define him by his disease. He is still whoever he was to you—friend, neighbor, co-worker. Remember what brought you to this point in your relationship—your shared history. Have you been his neighbor for ten years, his friend for twenty, his co-worker for fifteen? He is not just a person with cancer. He is an important person in your life. He may or may not want you to talk about the disease, but he will want to discuss the other interests you've shared.

"Hearing about cancer reminds me of another friend or family member's illness."

Each loss we face brings up memories of all our other losses. Mark, another group member, was feeling guilty about avoiding his friend Madeline, who had cancer. "It reminds me of when my father had it. I can't handle it," he said. "If she tells me about her experience, then I may have to open up and talk about *him*. I'm still not ready to discuss his five-year battle or those final months we spent together. I should have done more for him. I didn't tell him I loved him enough. I didn't..."

Mark assumed that calling Madeline would revive and magnify these old feelings, but her illness was going to bring them up whether he called her or not. By not calling her, he only added to his regrets the guilt of not contacting a good friend who needed him.

Finally he called her. "She didn't put any pressure on me to talk about my father. She only wanted to share her experiences."

A month later he reported a surprise. "The more I listened to her, the more it ended up helping me. By listening to Madeline, I began to understand what had happened with my father. Our talks have helped me more than they could ever have supported her."

"It makes me realize how vulnerable I am."

The recognition of vulnerability can raise fears as well. "If it could happen to her, then it could happen to me," you may think. Or: "I don't want to call him and hear the details of his father's cancer. My dad is close to his age."

These reactions can be very subtle. You may not even be aware you have them. Some relatives and friends have told me, "I felt awful, but I thought, 'At least it's not me.'" Others said, "This disease just scares me. I can't think about it or call my friend who has it."

We don't want to hear that something so horrible could happen. It upsets us not only because we care for the person, but because it makes us feel vulnerable. People our age don't get this sick. We want to believe we are going to live a long time. Hearing the news of someone else's illness challenges our beliefs about our mortality.

Jillian, a leukemia patient, found out that her friend Amy's breast cancer had returned five years after her doctor said she was cancer free: "I knew intellectually that we didn't even have the same type of cancer. We were two different people. Yet I didn't call her for weeks. The idea of any type of cancer returning terrified me."

A friend who doesn't call, so as not to hear the painful details, may think he will not be confronted by his own fears of the disease. In this assumption he may well be mistaken, and he may let down someone who needs to know that he is concerned.

"We're not that close."

Jillian added another reason for not calling Amy. "We aren't that close." I asked Jillian if they were close enough that Amy would be expecting her to call. Jillian replied, "Not only would she want me to call, her brother *asked* me to call her."

"I'm afraid I'll get in over my head."

If you aren't comfortable talking about the cancer or the emotions that accompany it, you can let your friend know that that's how you feel. You may also be uncomfortable because your friend really needs to talk to someone with experience—a counselor, doctor, clergyman, or another patient. In such a case you can say:

> "I don't know much about it. Let me look into it and
> see what I can find out."
> "I'm really not qualified to give you any answers. But I
> know of an agency that has professionals who may
> have some ideas about this."

If inexperience is not what is preventing you from talking to the person, then perhaps there are other reasons. Ask yourself:

> "What am I afraid of?"
> "What's the worst thing that could happen if I called?"
> "Do I have unresolved issues with this person?"
> "Am I afraid of discussing certain issues because I'm not
> sure how I feel toward the person?"
> "Am I so afraid of losing her that I can't talk about this
> with her or anyone else?"

If none of these reasons applies to you, you may want to talk over your resistance with someone you trust. Talking to someone who can be objective may make your issues more apparent and help you begin to resolve them.

Making Contact

Most of us have good intentions, and our friendships are valuable to us. But the longer you wait to contact someone who is ill, the harder it will ultimately be for *you*.

Sometimes the best way to do something you don't want to do is just to do it. Schedule a time to call when you will not be rushed. If you keep a daily to-do list, put it on the list and keep it there until you call.

If you still can't call your friend, turn to Chapter 5, "From the Goodness of Your Heart: 52 Gift Ideas." Giving a gift of time or an item your friend needs or will treasure can be as valuable as making a phone call. As Janet said, "The people who sent flowers or notes or provided help with the house meant as much to me as the people who called."

For the Primary Caregiver: Why You Can't Talk About It

Your barriers will be different from those of a friend, neighbor, or co-worker. You live with this person and you have an intimate connection with each other that has now been seriously altered. No matter how close you are, it's normal to be afraid to share what you are feeling. You may talk about what you are experiencing, medically or socially, but that can be much easier than talking about how this disease has affected you, how it has invaded every aspect of your life.

Perhaps you are so focused on her needs, you haven't even noticed how the illness is affecting you. Or maybe you feel you can't possibly tell her how scared you are or how helpless you feel.

Perhaps you've had marital problems, or maybe you are an adult child and this has brought up issues you never had to face. Or maybe you have always had problems with Dad, but now he is alone and depending on you to be his primary caregiver and so the dynamics are changing and you don't know how to react to them. You don't even know how you are feeling and so how can you talk with the person who needs you?

Whatever your situation, as the primary caregiver *you* are the one who has to take the brunt of the patient's emotions. And if the relationship has problems, as many do, these problems can be exacerbated by the stress you will both be under.

The situation does not get easier if you sweep your feelings under the rug, or try to ignore them or talk around them. However, before you try to discuss them with the patient, evaluate them by asking yourself if any of these comments reflect the way you feel:

"I don't want to talk about it with her, because I'm afraid she'll break down, and I just couldn't deal with that."

Jordan and Cinda had been married for thirty-nine years. They had four children spread across the country, who all considered themselves close to their parents. The family had endured a lot together, and they were proud of the way they had always supported each other. Yet when Cinda became ill, no one in the family was comfortable talking about her disease or what could happen to her.

"Initially my wife and I stayed away from each other," Jordan recalls. "This was out of character for us. The longer we stayed away, the harder it was to begin talking about the emotional aspects of the cancer. I was afraid if we talked about what we were feeling, she would start crying, and I wouldn't know what to do for her.

"Cinda finally confronted me because she was feeling isolated. The best thing we ever did was to talk about how sad we were about the loss of her health and what it meant to us. Then we cried together. Instead of its being the awful experience I expected, I felt completely comfortable with the tears."

Jordan's suggestion to loved ones is: "You aren't doing anyone any favors by avoiding tears, not even yourself. You aren't helping her, and you aren't proving that you are strong.

"If you avoid a topic because you think you can't talk about it, you will miss a wonderful opportunity to work it through together."

"It's his problem. He can't handle talking about his feelings."

Of course, *you* couldn't possibly be the one with the problem. Surely *he* is the one with the problem.

Before you decide someone else can't handle sharing feelings, ask him if that is really the case. It is easier to assume he can't talk about emotions than to risk bringing them up yourself. Maybe he can't handle them, but you won't know unless you initiate the conversation. You might say, "I really am struggling with my feelings. I wonder if you feel that way too." Or: "I'm really angry. How are you feeling about the changes that have occurred?"

"I can't talk about this because I'm afraid."

Ask yourself what are the five things you are most afraid of. Will not talking about these issues really make you less afraid?

"I'm too angry to talk, but I'm not sure why."

Serious illness rarely happens in an emotional vacuum. Our lives are complicated, and our emotions are often confusing—especially anger, because so many variables can trigger it. Let's say you arrive home at the end of the day. Your husband, who has cancer, says something that hits you the wrong way, and you lash out at him. You know that his comment isn't the real source of your reaction, only the trigger. The source is the way your boss spoke to you earlier in the day. You shoved your boss's remarks aside or even buried them somewhere. Your husband unwittingly reminded you of them by his comment.

Or let's say that for weeks you have been upset about your finances. Your wife mentions an argument that she had with the insurance company, over a bill that you didn't even know about. It triggers all of your anxious feelings about your financial situation. And you may be angry at your wife, for reasons you may not even be able to articulate.

Anger can also stem from childhood experiences, from emotional issues and patterns established long ago. When we are vulnerable, exhausted, and under tremendous stress, those issues creep back into our lives in ways that we may not understand. You may have spent years taking care of a parent, or you may have had the kind of relationship with a younger sibling in which you had to make all the decisions. You felt responsible, even overwhelmed. You vowed never to have such a relationship again. Yet now here you are taking care of someone else. Your loved one's illness can renew old resentments. How do you sort through these emotions? How do you even begin to understand them?

Ask Yourself Questions

Start by asking yourself, "What am I feeling right now?" Then write down ten things that bother you most, besides the disease. Then ask yourself what relationship reminds you of the one you are in now. When have you felt this way before? How did you deal with it then? How is this relationship different from that one?

You may not like the answers, but the more honest you are with yourself, the more you will get in touch with your feelings. You may also learn to separate the old issues from the present ones, or to understand better their impact on what is happening to you now.

When life's waters become turbulent, your life will feel out of control. We are taught to swim with a rough tide if it is pulling us out to sea—swimming against the tide can kill us. Going the other way is counterintuitive. How do you swim with your fears when your instincts are telling you to swim away from them?

First you must acknowledge that the emotions exist. Then you need to find constructive ways to incorporate them into your life.

Nothing Happens Easily

Dealing with your fears, as well as the rest of your feelings, will be a never-ending challenge. Certain emotions will turn up again and again. Others may be resolved for the first time in your life.

As you begin to work through some of your issues, however, you will grow more at ease in talking to your loved one. The sense that your emotions are overwhelming will recede. When you understand your underlying concerns and fears, you will feel more in control. It takes practice. Throughout this book you will find many coping techniques that you can use. The stories about how others have dealt with their emotions will help you to understand your feelings.

In the meantime, you still have to find a way to talk to your loved one. The next two chapters give you keys to compassionate conversation. The guidelines show you how to formulate your own ideas about what to say to someone facing a life-threatening illness.

Chapter 3

What Do I Say?:
How to Begin Talking When
You Don't Know What to Say

Lying there, he looked so small, so weary, aged beyond his years. His bed was tucked into a corner of the hospital wing, in what seemed to me a dark and depressing room. As a teenager, I did not care about my friend Jimmy's room or what he looked like. I just wanted to see him. Roland had had the idea of walking right by the sign on the door exclaiming FAMILY MEMBERS ONLY and right by the silent, angry glare of the nurse. He had strutted up to the metal railing by Jimmy's head, leaned over, taken his hand, and asked, "How are you holding up, my friend?" Jimmy glanced at the nurse. Then, as though instantly obliterating her from the room, he had cracked his notorious sexy smile and made some remark about doing well. Roland and I brought him up-to-date on the antics of our mutual friends. Jimmy was clearly captivated, and whatever pain I had seen when I entered this room vanished. We talked and talked about all the things we had shared—simple things, things I was positive that we would share again.

Toward the end of a conversation that is as clear today as it was back then, I remember thinking, "He looks more like himself now. Is that because we're here, or is it simply because someone, anyone, is talking to him, has invited him back into this world?" As we left, Jimmy was leaning on his left elbow, his right hand clutching his side of the bed as he laughed at Roland's last joke.

As teenagers, Roland and I probably did not say the "right things," and who knows if we acted the "right way," but the night Jimmy died, he gave my roommate that message: "Tell Elise I said thank you."

We all want to help a loved one or friend who is hurting, but knowing how is one of the hardest of challenges. Finding the most appropriate words is a common problem.

As you try to help your loved one, you may remember something that someone said to you when you were in pain, something that made you feel better, that gave you comfort. That person's kind and thoughtful words had a healing effect.

The suggestions that follow will help you bring comfort to your loved one. You probably won't say any of the phrases exactly as they appear here. We usually don't plan exactly what we are going to say— nor should we. It ought to come naturally. These suggestions are meant merely to serve as springboards to other ideas. Keeping them in mind can help you develop your own unique way of sharing your love.

If you don't agree with a suggestion, ignore it. You must decide what is the best way to help your loved one or friend. The key to building a loving relationship and giving of yourself is to communicate from the heart. The most important support you have to give is your presence and your willingness to listen and to help in any way you can. These actions are more important than any words you may say.

If you are a friend of the family, keep in mind that the rest of the family is hurting too. You can use most of these suggestions with family members as well as patients. I hope they enable you to talk to and understand the person you want to help.

1. Ask first.

> "I know my wife. I know exactly what she needs."
> "We'll clean this whole house, and Mom will be thrilled. Everyone wants help with cleaning."

Whatever the circumstance, whatever you want to do or discuss, the best principle to follow is: Ask first. Thousands of people have told me that they just wished their friends and relatives had asked them what they needed before trying to help. This is especially important for families under tremendous stress, whose circumstances change daily and whose disease has taken away so much of what they can control. They still need and want to control the things that make them feel worthwhile.

Janice, a thirty-six-year-old patient, told the members of her weekly support group, "I need to keep cooking dinner for my kids. It makes me feel like I am still me and still giving to them."

Nan, a forty-eight-year-old patient in the group, had a different view. "I'd give anything for someone to do the cooking," she laughed. "I'd rather do the shopping, but now my girls insist on doing it. They don't understand how good it makes me feel to get out and to shop for my family."

Jim, a single father, had a similar problem. "My older son came home and took over the cooking. It was a very nice gesture, but cooking relaxes me. I enjoy it. Now if he wanted to do the laundry, that'd be fine. I wish he'd ask what I need instead of assuming he knows."

Raney, a spouse, got upset about a social worker who assumed she knew what Raney needed. "The social worker tells me, 'We need to talk about plans for a hospice. You need to start thinking about it, and this is a good time.'

"I was shocked. How did she know what was a good time to talk?

If it was so important, why couldn't she just send me the brochures and say, 'Here's some information you may be interested in. If you want to talk about it, here's my number.'"

Jason was in a custody battle with his wife, who was a survivor of serious illness. A friend at work came into his office and gave him advice. "I think you need to talk about the fact that your wife could die soon," the man said.

Jason was furious. "How does he have any idea what I need to discuss, or if he's even the person I want to talk with about her possible death?"

In most situations the best approach is to assume you don't know what the person wants. Maybe the topic you want to discuss or the thing you want to do is a perfectly great idea, but you don't know what the person is going through or what she wants. And there is only one way to find out—ask her, before you plunge in with what you think she needs.

2. If your friend doesn't want to talk, it may have nothing to do with you.

If you have asked the person about the cancer and her answers are brief or evasive, she may not want to talk about it. The reasons could be any of several. She may not be ready. She may not be comfortable. Or she may have already chosen other people to talk with.

One client told me, "I have three people in whom I confide my feelings. I don't need to share them with anyone else."

The most important message you can convey is "I care about you. I want to listen if you need to talk. I'm here if and when you do." Beyond that, it is up to the person to take up your offer.

3. Be a student of the person you are trying to help.

Anne Turnage is the founder of CanCare, a program that provides volunteer counseling support. She trains volunteers, all of whom are cancer patients, to support others who are coping with cancer. She teaches them how to share their experiences, telling them: "No matter how much experience you have with this disease, approach each conversation as a student of the person you are trying to help. Each person has a unique set of experiences. You can't possibly know exactly what he is going through."

4. Don't plan your responses while you are listening.

How many times have you poured your heart out to someone, and when you are finished, the advice he gives you makes it obvious he hasn't heard most of what you've said? You know he cares about you and that he's only trying to help. Yet he was listening with his head, not his heart.

While the person is talking to you, don't mentally plan what you are going to say next. Focus on what the person is telling you. Pay attention to the tone of his voice, to his eyes, and to his body signals. These will give you important clues to what he is feeling and enable you to give him your full attention.

5. Become comfortable with silence.

Silence can be a time when people are thinking about their next statement or reflecting on the last one. Your silence can encourage your friend or loved one to expand on or rephrase a previous remark. It is a signal that you are listening. If you are peaceful, relaxed, and quiet, she is more likely to share information about herself than if you appear hurried, anxious, or preoccupied or if you cut her off, not allowing her time to gather her thoughts.

6. Take your cues from the person.

Let her lead the conversation and choose activities when you are together. Make suggestions, but don't push them.

7. Concentrate on being, not doing.

When you are talking to the person, she needs you to *be* with her, not to *do* anything for her. Your presence speaks for itself. The most important job you have is to listen to her troubles, not to fix them.

8. *Refrain from offering advice until you are asked.*

Do you really have the best answer? Most likely you don't. Answers are often complex and beyond our reach. Jumping in with unsolicited advice is a way of taking control over a situation. Encouraging someone to search for his own answers, by contrast, empowers him to take control himself. You are there to support your friend or loved one, not to supply him with a solution to his problem.

He mostly needs to vent his feelings while you listen. By sharing his thoughts, he'll discover the answer himself.

When people want your ideas, they will usually ask for them. Before you give advice, read the rest of these guidelines. They will enable you to offer advice in ways that are helpful, not harmful.

9. *Make suggestions without expecting the person to use them.*

If the person does solicit your advice, share your suggestions, but do not expect him to accept all of your ideas. He is gathering different viewpoints. He will ultimately use only the ones that are right for him.

10. *Be empathetic, not sympathetic.*

Sister Alice Potts, from M. D. Anderson Cancer Center, approaches families with empathy, not with sympathy. "When I'm being *sympathetic,* I feel responsible for others. I use lots of *shoulds* and *oughts* and waste my energy. I want to fix the person, make him better. But I'm just going in circles, like a dog chasing its tail. I never reach my goal. I never accomplish what I want to because I cannot fix anyone.

"When I'm being *empathetic,* I don't take away the person's power. People need to believe they can handle things, that they have control.

Empathy conveys that I believe they can regain control. When I approach them this way, I'm more loving and more relaxed, because I'm there to support them, not to control them."

People coping with any disease don't want sympathy. They want to be heard, understood, and accepted. They realize that you don't know exactly how they are feeling, but it is helpful if you try to understand the situation from their point of view.

Ask yourself how you would feel if this happened to you. You might react differently. Thinking about the question may give you some insight into what they are feeling.

11. Listen to what is under the surface.

Bang—your mother-in-law slams the table with her fist. "I'm not angry," she says, gritting her teeth.

Your child is standing in a corner, shredding Kleenex and wiping her face. Her eyes are red. "This doesn't upset me at all," she says.

Sometimes what is under the surface isn't as obvious as it is in these cases.

During one of my family support group sessions, Sandy, a forty-five-year-old mother of three, complained about her little sister. "Lynn isn't helping me care for our father, who is battling prostate cancer," said Sandy. "I've called Lynn and suggested ways she could get involved. But she rarely agreed to do anything, and when she did agree to help, she didn't follow through.

"You know," Sandy added, "she's never there when you need her. Why can't she just be like my brother? He's always willing to do whatever I ask. He knows how hard this is on all of us. He never complains."

Over the next few weeks, the group members offered Sandy suggestions to get Lynn involved. Nothing Sandy tried worked. Each week she became more frustrated.

A month later Sandy realized what was really upsetting her. "I miss my sister," she told the group, "and I wish I had her to go through this with. I really don't care how much she does. I just wish we could talk about my father, like we did when he had a heart attack a few years back. We were so close then. We've always been close, but this illness has torn us apart, and I don't know why. I'd be happy if we could just talk."

The group realized that beneath Sandy's anger lay pain. It was the relationship with her sister that she was missing, not the help. Once Sandy understood what was under the surface, she called Lynn.

Lynn surprised Sandy when she said she had wanted to call her for weeks but was afraid Sandy would just ask her to do things for their parents. Lynn wasn't ready to get involved. All that she wanted was to talk to her big sister.

12. Be honest with each other and with the people who can help.

Sheryl dutifully accompanied her husband, Roger, to every doctor's visit, even though his behavior in the waiting room upset her. She later said to me, "Roger tells me in tremendous detail, moaning while he talks, with emphasis on every pain, what he is feeling. Then he struts into the doctor's office with this huge smile on his face. He tells the man, 'I'm fine, just a few aches, Doc.'"

One day Sheryl couldn't accept his dishonesty anymore. She hated what it did to her. "I was being dishonest myself by not saying anything, and that tore me apart."

After months of deception Sheryl finally said, "You know, Roger, this bothers me. I'm really uncomfortable with having information about your health that you don't share with the doctor. I'm worried he won't be able to help you if he doesn't know what's wrong. How will he know what to do if you don't tell him your symptoms? I would feel better about going to these visits if you would share what you tell me with the doctor."

Sheryl confronted Roger by sharing her own feelings, not by

attacking him. Sometimes, you will have to take an active role to maintain honesty in the person's relationship with the physician.

Roger agreed that his doctor should know his symptoms, but he couldn't tell the doctor to his face what was wrong. An organized, practical engineer, he could, however, write it down. So he listed his symptoms and handed the list to the physician at the beginning of their next visit. One of those "minor" symptoms was actually a red flag that alerted the doctor to change the treatment immediately.

Eight years later, Roger tells anyone who will listen, "Be honest with your doctor." Whenever Sheryl hears this, she always smiles.

13. Give realistic encouragement.

Eugene, the forty-one-year-old cancer client from Chapter 2 who made his friends laugh, once told me that during chemotherapy, "the people who drove me crazy were the ones who had stupid, silly, you-can-spot-them-a-mile-away grins. They acted like one-person cheerleading squads.

"I did have a positive attitude and I love to joke, but I was realistic too. I wanted people to be hopeful and encouraging—but not only about a cure."

There are so many other things to be encouraging about, including that when someone is ill, she will still have good days and be free of pain; that her family will have the strength to manage her cancer; that each day she will find events that are special and meaningful; that she will develop or strengthen her faith; and that she and her family will continue to build their dreams and find peace in whatever happens.

Eugene continued: "I had stage-four metastatic cancer. It's the worst kind. So when someone acted as if it would be easy to cure or everything was going to be all right, that upset me. Either they didn't understand, or they didn't want to acknowledge how serious my situation was. Even if they couldn't do that, they could have given me encouragement in the more practical and simpler areas of my life."

14. *Touch the person on the arms or hands when he is talking, and give him a hug when you begin and/or end a visit.*

Sometimes a gesture offers comfort better than words. The human spirit thrives on feeling connected to others. Touching is one of the best ways to let your loved one or friend know you care. Be aware of body language, though—if he pulls away, it is a sign he isn't comfortable with that kind of closeness.

15. *Maintain a comfortable posture and eye contact.*

Have you ever talked to people who do not look you in the eye, who fidget, or who look like they have a more important place to be? It makes you feel as if they aren't interested in you or are in a hurry to leave.

It's hard for your loved one or friend to think you are listening if you are looking around the room. Lack of eye contact can be taken as a sign of indifference or even as a put-down. Looking directly at the person who is speaking shows you are paying attention.

Unfold your arms as much as possible. Sit back in your chair, and get comfortable. Settle in as if you were staying for a little while, even if you are staying for only a few minutes. If your back is rigid and you cross your arms over your chest, you appear to be closing yourself off.

Leaning toward the person speaking and occasionally nodding your head or interjecting comments (ah huh, umm, hmm) shows you are listening. You appear interested in what the person is saying.

16. *Don't be afraid to say the word cancer.*

As Bob Davis advised in *I Have Cancer, This Is What You Can Do,* a Cancer Counseling brochure for family members, "Say the word *cancer*." He explains: "Fred Rogers of *Mister Rogers* once said of talking to children about sensitive matters, 'If it's human, it's mentionable.' If this advice is good enough for children, why shouldn't it be good enough for adults? Try saying things like, 'What did the doctor say about the cancer on your last visit?'

"Most people who come in contact with me avoid asking me direct questions. They choose instead to keep the conversation away from illness. You need not trivialize the issue, nor do you need to be maudlin. Just don't avoid the subject."

17. Sometimes it's best to begin with the medical facts.

In the early stages of the illness, it may be helpful to ask the person about the medical facts of the disease. She may not be ready to talk about her feelings yet, either because she is in shock, or because she has chosen only a few people to discuss her feelings with, or because she doesn't want to discuss her feelings with anyone. If this is the case, she may find it less threatening to discuss facts. In fact, repeating the facts to you may help her deal with the diagnosis.

At the beginning of my weekly support groups, members would share facts: what happened at the most recent doctors' visit; the side effects of a treatment; the latest cancer research; a specific doctor; a resource they had discovered; how their kids were doing. Exchanging information was a way group members could catch up with one another, reaffirm their relationships, and break the initial tension. It was less threatening than discussing emotions, since it required less trust. Once the group members realized that the others were interested in their medical stories, they were more willing to open up and delve into their feelings.

Your friend or loved one may be evaluating how comfortable you are with the diagnosis. She may bring up the subject of feelings spontaneously when she thinks you are comfortable with the facts.

Once she starts talking about feelings to you, you can guide the conversation toward feelings in future encounters. However, if you try once or twice to bring up something emotional and she stays with the facts, return to the facts. At that moment she doesn't want to share her feelings. It doesn't mean she will never discuss them with you again. At another time she may be more open.

Be alert for signals that she doesn't want to discuss her feelings. She may change the subject or give short, curt answers to questions. There may also be times when you are not comfortable discussing feelings. In any of these cases, you can ask questions about medical topics, such as:

> "What tests were there?"
> "What kind of treatment are they recommending?"
> "How is the treatment progressing?"

18. Say how you feel first.

Stating your own feelings may be a good way to open up a conversation if it is one of your parents who is ill or if it is someone who tends to be protective of other people's feelings. Parents especially may not want to burden you, or they may be uncomfortable talking to you about their illness. For such reasons, many adult children do not get important information about their parents' disease.

When you state how you feel, you may want to express the pain you are experiencing as a result of not understanding what is going on. Most parents will want to make you feel better and will at least give you general information about their medical condition. You could say, "I love you. I'm really upset. I need to know what you are feeling." Or: "I'm so upset, and I love you. It's hard not knowing what is going on. Can you tell me about it?" Or you could share your love first: "Mom, I love you. You are so important to me, and right now I feel cut off from you. I know this is hard for you to discuss, but I feel helpless not knowing what is going on."

19. Don't cover up your feelings.

Don't say: "I'm not worried. I know everything is going to be fine."

Say: "I'm scared too. This is a serious operation. But I'm going to be here for you. We'll get through this together."

Eugene explains, "People didn't have to pretend there was nothing wrong with me. They didn't have to hide their feelings. But they did.

Sometimes I felt sorrier for them than for me. What I really appreciated was when they told me they were scared, mad, or worried. Their empathy made me feel as though they understood what I was going through."

If your loved one is about to undergo major surgery, be honest if you are scared. Then tell him how you feel about him, not just his disease:

> "I'm worried about the scars too, and I'm upset that you have to go through this. But all I really care about is keeping you well, and to me those scars represent that the doctors are going to get rid of the cancer, that they can treat this."
>
> "I don't like the scars either, but I want you well, and that's more important than any scars."
>
> "I hate that you have to live with any scars. I wish you didn't have them. But I'd rather see them than lose you."
>
> "It's not your body I'm in love with, it's you, your heart, your soul, how you act, how you laugh, how you are with the kids, and how you treat me."

He will appreciate your honesty. You may be surprised to find that your ability to be open and honest will become a catalyst to more revealing and intimate conversations and to a stronger relationship.

20. Help the person clarify her feelings.

He says: "I'm really feeling scared about the chemotherapy. I'm not even sure it will work."

Don't say: "You shouldn't feel scared. I heard they can control the side effects. Look on the bright side—this time next year you'll be cancer free."

"You *should* be glad—fifteen years ago they couldn't even treat this."

"You should be glad they caught it when they did."

"You should be happy, at least it's not (and then mention a disease you think is worse, like leprosy)."

Say: "It must be scary waiting to find out if the treatment will work."

"It must be hard going through this treatment and not knowing if it will work."

21. If he brings up feelings, stay with the feelings.

There are simple ways to guide the conversation and keep it focused on the person's feelings.

Patient: "The chemotherapy starts next week. I'm worried about how my kids are going to handle this if something goes wrong."

Don't say: "Well, at least the treatments only last a week at a time."

Say: "It must be scary facing the treatments and not being able to tell them how it will work out."

"It must be so hard worrying about how the kids will do if something goes wrong. Have you thought about what you are going to tell them before you go in? Have you shared your concerns? Have you told them you're worried?"

22. Don't be judgmental; accept and support what they are feeling.

Unless you have been through it yourself, you can never know how you would react if you were in this situation. People react to illness in individual ways. There is no right way. Your friend or loved one may not be acting as you would, but his reaction is affected by his unique experiences, attitudes, and expectations. For example, if he says, "This really scares me," don't say, "You have nothing to be afraid of," or "You shouldn't be scared, you're in good hands," or "You'll do just fine, don't worry."

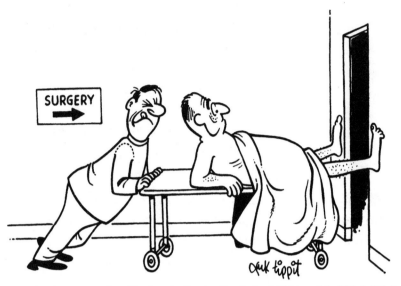

SURGERY →

Instead, let him know you accept and support him.

Say: "This must not seem fair at all, especially now, but I'm going to do everything I can to help you through this."

"I'll never know exactly what you are feeling, but if we talk about it, I can do my best to understand and be here for you."

"I can only begin to imagine how hard this must be. I'm going to be here for you. I'll support you in whatever ways you think will be most helpful."

23. When the question is "why," the answer is "I don't know."

Your friend may ask you why she got sick, or how it could have happened to her now. "I never did anything wrong. Why did I get this?" she may ask. Or: "I thought I was in perfect health—how could this happen?"

To questions like these, you probably don't have the answers. There may never be answers. Yet the patient's need to ask the questions, to struggle with them, and to try to make sense of them, is real. If answers exist, they are very personal and complex.

If your friend or loved one asks these questions, say, "I don't understand why this is happening," or simply acknowledge that it is hard to make sense of it all.

24. Don't correct the person. Ask for clarification when you don't understand.

Don't say: "But last week when you told me about the chemotherapy, you said..."

"No, that's the wrong way to look at this."

"Don't feel that way—you should be happy because the tests were negative."

Say: "I'm not sure what you mean."

"If I understood what you just said, then do you mean..."

As he clarifies his thoughts, it will give both of you a better understanding of the situation.

25. Ask questions that require more than a yes-or-no answer.

Ask questions that spark conversation or require detailed answers. Such questions will give the person a reason to extend her thoughts.

Don't ask: "Are you sad?"

Ask: "How are you feeling? Have you tried or heard about anything new to control the pain?"

Don't ask: "How was your day?"

Ask: "Tell me about your mother's visit. What did you do? Did it go as well as you'd thought it would?"

26. Let him finish what he is saying.

If you are in a rush or you are excited and want him to know you understand, you might interrupt him before he finishes his thoughts. You probably mean well, but it comes across as disregard for his feelings or lack of interest in what he is saying. Be patient and listen.

27. *Validate what she is saying by not changing the topic when she finishes speaking.*

When we are uncomfortable with someone else's pain or anger or confusion, it is normal to want to make her feel better by saying things that we think will help. After your loved one completes a thought, you may want to say, "It will be all right," or "Everything is going to work out," or "Now that we've talked about that, let's focus on the positive."

A British researcher from the University of Manchester, Dr. Peter Maguire, has observed that health care professionals and family members often change the topic this way unwittingly. The loved one or person with cancer says, "I am really scared," and the nurse or doctor responds, "Yes, but how's your leg today?"

Changing the subject invalidates what the person has been trying to tell you. You may be perceived as trivializing her emotions, or attempting to talk her *out* of her feelings instead of *through* them. Stay on the topic she is discussing.

28. *Pay attention to the person's moods.*

Often when I am talking with a client about cancer, I can see them pulling away from the subject. They become evasive or abrupt, or they sound as though they wish the conversation would end. They stop telling me details.

They may have already shared more than they cared to, or they may simply have said enough for one day. Perhaps they've changed gears and want to discuss a different topic. At that point I disengage from the conversation or change the subject, out of respect for their feelings.

Throughout a conversation with your loved one or friend, you can ask, "Do you want to keep on talking about this?" Or: "Are you comfortable talking about this now?"

If she doesn't seem comfortable, find a polite way to say, "It might be a bad day to talk about this." Or: "Do you want to talk about it now, or would another time be better?"

29. It's okay to cry.

"God didn't give you tear ducts for nothing," notes Sister Alice Potts. Nurse Mary Hughes points out, "We never apologize when we laugh. Why should we say we're sorry when we cry?"

Gentle tears show the person that you care for him. They also convey the message, "I am comfortable with your expression of sadness, with your tears."

Sometimes the person will cry and then apologize. Let him know he doesn't have to say he is sorry: "Please don't apologize for crying. I'd worry if you *weren't* upset. I know I am. It's a natural reaction." Or you can say, "Sometimes tears are the best way to express your emotions."

30. Avoid clichés at all costs.

Don't say: "Things could be worse," or "Time will take care of everything," or "It's all for the best." Such comments trivialize the situation.

31. Keep private conversations private.

The person is talking to you—not to your friend, not to your neighbor, not to your spouse, not to your mother. Your conversation is an intimate sacred trust. To repeat it to anyone would destroy that trust.

32. Be careful when you share.

Some people don't want to hear about someone else who had cancer. It may even be offensive. To them, the most irritating words you can say are, "Well, Jane had the same cancer, and she . . ."

Others don't mind hearing stories if you leave out gory details. One client said, "The last thing I needed to hear was how awful someone else's experience was. It didn't make me feel better."

Still other people want to hear other medical stories. One person said, "I want to hear about someone else who survived the same treatment, or about a person who is alive five years later with my type of disease. Those stories keep me going."

Before you share your experience, always ask the person if he wants to hear it. Better yet, wait until he says, "Do you know of anyone else who has been through this?" Or: "What happened to you when you went through it?"

If your friend or loved one asks you to share your own experiences, do so only if you are comfortable. Anne Turnage advises: "When you begin your story, say, 'Everyone is so different. No two people will have the exact same disease or experience. No two people react to the treatment the same way. No one can predict exactly how you will react, but maybe my story can give you some idea of what to expect.'"

Do not say your experiences were better, harder, or more profound. Never compare. Your story is just your version of what happened to you. You may have the exact same disease. The person may even be on the same medication as you were. But your reactions may be completely different. You can always give him educational materials on the side effects of a treatment or refer him to his doctor for this information.

Your job is to focus on the positive aspects of the disease—the lessons you learned from it, the changes you have made, the improvements in your life, the funny things that happened, and the people you met along the way. Share these inspirational stories.

33. Respect the person's spirituality.

Religious beliefs are very private. Although they are central to some individuals' entire approach to coping with this disease, they are still personal. My own faith is the foundation of how I deal with all aspects of my life. It is a faith, however, that I would discuss in depth only with certain people.

Wait until the person asks for your views before you discuss them. You may think you know her beliefs, but she may have changed drastically.

If the subject of religion arises, ask her how she wants to address it. She may want to share her beliefs with you, or she may want you to pray with her or for her, or she may want you to read passages from the Bible.

If you are uncomfortable talking about religious beliefs, say, "I don't know myself, but I can find someone [a chaplain, nun, or rabbi] with experience in this area."

Above all, be sure *not* to make statements like the following, which have been mentioned repeatedly by my clients as ones they wish never to hear: "God only gives you what you can handle." "It's God's will." "It's in God's hands."

Leanne had difficulty with statements like these. "I had very deep faith," she told me, "and I knew we would come out of this, but I needed to find my own way with my religion. It's too private for someone to be talking about with me. But I don't mind if someone tells me, 'I will say a prayer for you,' or 'I'm praying for you or keeping you in my prayers.' This is doing something they believe in."

Bridgett, the wife of a client, got really mad when she heard about God's will. "I don't believe any of this is God's will. How does anyone know what God's will is?" she demanded.

An adult daughter of a man who was dying had another view. "Right now, I'm really having trouble with my faith. The last thing I want anyone doing is preaching to me."

Claude, another client, suggested an alternative to the spiritual clichés. "I really appreciated it when people said they would pray for me or mailed me copies of inspirational passages from the Bible," he said. "It was something they could actively do to support me. I could read these stories on my own or ignore them. There wasn't any pressure. All other religious gestures or comments felt like clichés or judgments, and I found them to be turnoffs."

34. Tell your friend or loved one how much you love him.

"I love you. You are one of the most important people in my life. I cherish our relationship. My life is what it is because you are part of it."

Now is the time, more than any other, to let your friend or loved one know how important he is to you. Tell him what he does that is special, how he affects you, what your life is like because of him, what you've learned from him, and how incredibly valuable he is to you.

A serious illness presents you with opportunities to express your feelings. It is a good time to share how much your loved one means to you and what a difference he makes in your life. The response you get after you share these feelings will probably inspire you to continue to share your love, not only with the patient but with others in your life as well.

35. Let her know you will be there in the future.

If your loved one or friend doesn't want to discuss the cancer now, accept it. "I understand," you can say. "But I want you to know I'm here for you and available if you ever want to discuss it in the future."

36. Be yourself.

It's important for you to be yourself. Don't worry about saying the exact words or behaving in the precise manner described in these guidelines.

You may get nervous, or interrupt, or say something you wish you hadn't. That's normal for anyone in a new or stressful situation. Keep trying to be supportive. Your compassion and willingness to learn will come across. And that's what she really needs from you—your love, your compassion, and your presence.

The next chapter gives you guidelines on more complicated issues—issues about hope, humor, and dying. These topics usually arise at least a few weeks after the initial diagnosis. Depending on your circumstances, however, you may be discussing them sooner.

A friend once said to me, "I hope you tell your readers that there isn't a simple formula for everyone, but there can be guidelines." Your situation is unique. The ideas presented here can stimulate your thoughts and show you the different ways your loved one *may* be feeling. Adapt the suggestions to your situation. Whenever you are not sure about what you are doing, ask the person: "What's the best way I can help? What can I say that would make you feel better?"

Chapter 4

Along the Way:
Keys to the Tougher Conversations

"I'm not always easy to be around," said Eliza. "I can drive even the calmest person crazy. I realize this disease is tough on those who care about me. But I'm doing the best I can.

"They're afraid of losing me, but they will only lose one person. I'm dealing with losing everyone and everything I know. If they can just be understanding, I may just stick around and pester them longer than the doctors say I will."

After Eliza was diagnosed with metastatic bone cancer, the doctors had given her three months to live. Tacked onto their predictions were several warnings: She would probably experience severe pain, and she should give up traveling.

Eliza joined a one-year couples support group that I was leading, and at the end of the year she fully expected to go on to my next group. She had every intention of proving the doctors wrong. She did finish that group, and the next one. Meanwhile, she and her son traveled to three countries. She and her husband, Shane, made trips to two countries and six states.

The day before she died, almost four years later, Eliza took her third pain pill. Once during a support group session, she turned to Shane and said, "If you do these things [i.e., treat her in the ways described below], then I can keep going. But first I'll have to spend my IRA, your IRA, and maybe some savings." He gladly spent the money, and Eliza kept her word.

Eliza wanted to be treated in a certain way not only by Shane but by her co-workers, friends, and family members. Shane and her son wanted others to act toward them in much the same way. You can follow these guidelines, like the ones in Chapter 3, when you are supporting patients or loved ones. They address some of the more complex issues that may arise.

1. Help the person develop hope without ignoring other emotions.

Don came to a support group I was leading two days after he was rushed to the hospital. "I was very close to dying," he said.

"Last night, as we were pulling away from the medical center onto an overpass, my wife pointed out the sun lowering its reflection across the towering buildings, outlining the Houston skyline. Vivid blues, soothing oranges, and fiery reds draped themselves across what were once, to me, only concrete structures. I'd driven over that overpass a million times, but I never noticed how spectacular the view was.

"My wife understands that I still need to talk about how serious my illness is. I still need all of you to let me rant, rave, and rail against this disease. But every day I now look forward to many things I never noticed or appreciated before."

Help your friend or loved one discover hope and focus on the positive aspects of life. Yet, don't ignore bad feelings in the process. Have you ever told someone how awful your day was, then after you told him, you felt great? Just telling him relieved a burden for you. If the person had cut you off because you weren't being positive, your bad day would not have disappeared. You would still have the negative feelings and you wouldn't have anyone to share them with.

Hope doesn't have to be focused only on living longer or finding a cure. People can learn to hope that their experience will help others, or that they will enjoy special times with their family, achieve a short-term goal, learn from their experience, or notice something they had missed before.

2. Keep your sense of humor, and welcome hers.

One of the greatest gifts you can share is your wit—your sense of humor and your stories. If humor doesn't come naturally to you, then share a funny experience about one of your children or pets—your cat's latest antics, or your child's most recent escapade.

Watching a lighthearted movie or comedy together is another way to share humor. Playing a board game, cards, or a computer game can also create a lighthearted atmosphere.

Humor is an important component in healing and creating a sense of well-being. But be careful not to hide behind it. Pay attention to your own reasons for joking. Take your cues about humor from the person and respect her need to joke and make fun of things.

If someone who is sick cracks morbid jokes or makes fun of the hospital staff or anyone else, she may actually be trying to protect her feelings. She may also be trying to release the tension and defuse some of the intensity of the situation. Do not criticize her. Humor can be one of the most productive outlets, one of the best techniques for managing a tremendous amount of stress. Once she has laughed about a situation and released her tension, she can gain a clearer understanding of it.

3. Encourage the person to maintain dignity and independence.

Sometimes it's hard to avoid taking over your loved one's life. If you hover over him or try to take on all of his responsibilities, including ones he can still fulfill, you rob him of the opportunity to feel good about himself. Give him the room to discover what he can and cannot do.

4. Say more than "You look great."

Throughout the next weeks and months, you may run into someone coping with cancer at the office or at the supermarket, or you will visit her at her home. The first thing you may think is that she looks good. Or maybe she doesn't, but you think telling her she does will make her feel better. Or maybe you think that considering what she's going through, she does look great or better than could be expected.

To tell someone who feels awful that she looks great invalidates how she is feeling. These few words can place a tremendous burden on her, implicitly instructing her to act as if she felt good. Even though you mean well, your friend can interpret your words to mean that you don't understand the enormity of what she is facing.

If she really does look good and you want to tell her so, then add, "But how are you doing?" Acknowledge that she may not be feeling well.

5. Discuss your fears without being morbid.

Lisa was three weeks into her chemotherapy. In a support group where clients were talking about their fears, she said, "My friend Debbie told me I was the best friend she ever had. She said she was sure I was going to beat this, but she couldn't help being scared she would lose me.

"When she revealed her fears, I felt she really cared about me. Her honesty made me feel safe enough to talk about my own fears. Everyone else made statements to me that made it clear I had to be brave and that I shouldn't talk or think about anything negative.

"With Debbie, I felt like I could share my worst fears and be honest about how serious my illness was. Opening up and sharing my negative feelings made them less overwhelming. They weren't so bad once I could express them."

6. Be patient.

When my mother was having a hard time talking about the pain she was in as a result of nerve damage from her surgery, someone told me, "Be patient." I remember thinking that if I had any patience at all, it would be much more than a virtue.

It isn't always easy to be patient when you're stressed out, overworked, exhausted, and worried about your loved one. As best you can, try to have patience with yourself and the people around you.

People in this situation may be upbeat one moment and depressed or crying the next. Some days they will have a lot of energy, and other days none. Patients experiencing chronic pain, receiving chemotherapy, or recovering from surgery may have to endure weeks, months, and even years of fatigue or physical pain. My mother would play golf one day, walking eighteen holes while carrying her golf bag. A week later she'd leave the dinner table because she was in too much pain to sit in the chair.

Your friend or loved one may be interested in every word you have to say on one day and barely be able to concentrate on another. She may pour her heart out to you during one conversation but seem uninterested in the same topic later.

These reactions are normal. Be patient with yourself and others when this happens.

7. Fulfill simpler wishes.

If your friend tells you he wants something and you can give it to him, by all means do so. One woman said, "All I wanted was a card when I finished chemotherapy—a two-dollar card saying 'Congratulations.'

"I asked my husband and son to buy one, but they never did. My husband didn't want to jinx my good fortune. My son just didn't do it. I don't ask for a lot, but please give me the smaller things in life. They are important to me, even if they aren't to you."

8. *Remain open-minded.*

People may feel one way one moment and another way the next. Before you judge your friend's overall condition, wait and see how he is over a period of time. If you assume you know what he needs too quickly, you may do things that aren't helpful.

9. *There's more than one viewpoint on denial.*

Some people refuse to go to a doctor even though they are sick— they lose a significant amount of weight, they cough up a storm, or they sleep all the time. Yet they refuse to go. Others go through diagnostic tests and begin treatment, then quit because they don't believe they have cancer or they think it can go away on its own. These people are putting their health at risk. Medical personnel have to confront this type of denial because it's life-threatening.

But someone who refuses treatment and understands the repercussions of his decision is not in denial. He has made an educated choice not to undergo treatment. His choice may be different from what you might have wished. You will have to learn to respect and accept his choice, however, even though you disagree. No other stance will support him, even if you think it will.

Another kind of denial can be functional, as it was in Naomi's case.

When Naomi joined my couples group, she was young and vibrant, an avid golf and tennis player. Introducing herself, she told the group, "I have a rare form of cancer. I've gone to four major medical centers. They had nothing to offer me. My husband, Pete, and I have researched alternative treatments. We've gone to clinics in the United States, France, and Mexico. I've had enough. I've stopped treatment and do not want to discuss medical alternatives anymore."

Pete jumped in. "But I can't give up. I want to talk about continuing treatment. Naomi is in denial. If she doesn't want to discuss it anymore, it's because she doesn't realize we still have options."

The fact, however, was that Naomi wanted to enjoy whatever time she had left. She had gone as far with medical treatment as she was able to go. She fully understood the consequences of her decision.

During another session, one that Naomi did not attend, Dr. Decker, my co-leader in the group, told Pete, "Naomi probably isn't in denial, but if she is, she needs it to survive. Her denial allows her to get up in the morning and function throughout the day."

By focusing on each day and not just on her impending death, Naomi was able to live life to its fullest. If Pete had continued to push her, the quality of their life together would have been destroyed. And she had told him more than once, "All I want is to be with you and enjoy what we do have, not search for what we don't."

Eventually Pete agreed. He learned to accept and respect Naomi's wishes.

A few months later Pete called me and said he wanted to share his feelings with Naomi before she died. We discussed a gentle but honest way to do this. He would focus on his feelings, his love and his sadness, using statements beginning with "I feel" instead of "You did this or that."

The next day he shared his hopes, his dreams, and his regrets and said good-bye, leaving none of his feelings unsaid. Naomi listened quietly, and then she spoke: "I'm sorry this has been so hard for you. I wish it could have been another way. Thank you, Pete, for being honest with me, for respecting me, and for empowering me to live my life the way I needed to. I believe we've had times that were so full of joy this last year because you continued to support me without trying to control me. I will always love you, and I know you will carry me in your heart."

After they talked, Pete left Naomi with the nurse and went out to do some errands. An hour later, she died peacefully.

10. Ask the person if he wants someone to coordinate information.

Some families get inundated with calls and questions and talk about the person with cancer. I have heard many frustrated family members exclaim, "If one more person mentions the cancer, I'll..." If this is how your family feels, look for one person in the patient's office, congregation, or neighborhood to update everyone else about what is happening with him.

If you, as a friend or co-worker, become the point person, share only what the family has told you they want others to know. Keep a list of the people you have spoken to, so the family is aware of who has been contacted.

If you are not the point person, respect the family's choice to relegate this task to someone else. If there is something you want to know about the illness, ask the point person first. You can still make yourself available and be supportive in many other ways. If the family has also asked the point person to assign chores, projects, and anything else they want done, then ask the point person how you can help.

11. Establish times to call.

Some people telephone a patient or their family in the afternoons, when they have visitors. It is more helpful to find out when they are alone. But if you just say to the person "Call me if you need me," it only adds one more burden and it sounds insincere. Instead, set a specific time to call. If you schedule a time to talk and follow through by calling at that time, she will appreciate your consideration.

That doesn't mean you should call every day. You can ask her how often she would like you to call. Some people really need and want their friends' daily support. Others feel bombarded by well-meaning friends and neighbors. They would prefer you called less often.

If you are calling for the first time, you can say:

> "I wanted to see how you were doing. When is the best time to talk?"
>
> "Do you have time to talk now? If not, I'd be happy to call back when it's more convenient."
>
> "Did I catch you at a good time? If you're busy, I can call back later."
>
> "Please be honest with me about this. If you need me to call every day, I would be happy to. Please let me know what will help you the most."

If you call and get her answering machine, leave a message so she can call you back at her convenience. If she has company, doesn't feel well, needs to be alone, or is in the middle of doing something, your message will let her know you care.

Sometimes friends of the family will complain that they always reach the answering machines. But when people's lives are turned upside down, they often need quiet evenings, moments away from the chaos. They need silence, time to regroup and be alone. One way they gain control over the incredible demands placed on their time is to screen their phone calls and set aside a specific time to talk on the phone.

12. *Keep your visits short, unless the patient asks you to stay longer.*

If you visit your friend at home or in a hospital room, he may be overwhelmed, in pain, or exhausted. Let him know that whatever makes him comfortable is what is most important to you.

Most likely, he will be glad to see you, but watch for signals that he is becoming tired. You might suggest, "Tell me when it's time to take a nap, or when you're getting tired." Or: "Time just gets away from me. Let me know when you're tired."

Some patients want you to spend longer periods of time with them—hours sitting quietly, reading, or watching television together. If you are visiting for several hours, ask him how he would like to spend the time with you.

13. *Avoid saying things that hospital patients would rather not hear.*

In a brochure printed by Churches of Christ Medical Center Chaplaincy, Chaplain Virgil Fry lists a number of statements that hospital patients would rather not hear:

"I've just got a second to say hi."
"Did you know massive doses of vitamins could have prevented that?"

"Hospital food is always terrible."

"I hope you appreciate all the trouble I went to to find this place."

"It sure is hot in here. I'll tell the nurse to adjust the thermostat."

"At least you're getting a break from the kids."

"I can't believe I had to pay to park just to see you."

"I've never seen you with your hair not combed."

"I'd give you a hug, but I'm afraid I'd get sick."

"I'd have come sooner, but I didn't know you were this bad."

"At least you don't have as many stitches as my grandmother did."

"Eat. Don't you want to get out of the hospital?"

"Isn't what you had done considered minor surgery?"

"My cousin had the same surgery, and he never even took a pain pill."

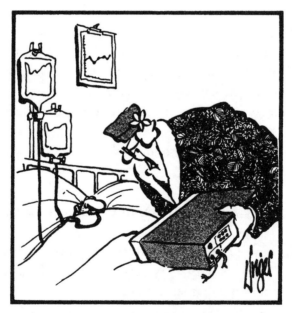

"Show me what to press if I want to record a movie after I've gone to bed."

14. Be considerate when visiting a patient who is in bed.

If you have ever been ill and in bed, you may have had some uncomfortable moments with visitors. Have you ever had people visit you and stand in the door as if they're ready to leave, or plop down on your feet, practically pushing you out of the bed?

If the patient is sitting, then sit down yourself. If he is standing, then stand. If she is in bed, ask, "Where is the best place for me to sit?"

Clara, a proud sixty-eight-year-old woman, told me as she lay in a hospital bed, "I've never set foot in a hospital." Then her shoulders sagged, and she fiddled with a stack of Kleenex. "I'm frightened. I feel so alone here."

Sitting up, she pointed toward the door: "My sister just makes it worse. She stands right there, one foot just outside my room, with her arms folded. She yanks her head around when anyone walks by. Doesn't want to miss a thing. I feel even more isolated when she's here than when she's not."

In contrast, Stanley, a usually reserved retired airline pilot, had a visitor who made him feel cared for. "I always appreciated my doctor. This tiny man, with no hair and squinty eyes, sits down on the edge of the bed when he talks to me. He pushes his glasses up on his head and lays his chart down, explaining every detail of my care, as though he's memorized it. I never feel as if he's rushed, even when he's only here for a few minutes."

Dr. Judy Headley, a member of the Nursing Oncology Society and an associate professor at the University of Texas Nursing School, adds, "Remember, even if someone is in the hospital, you are a guest in her room. Resist the urge to move furniture or plants unless you are asked to do so."

15. Be open to conversation about death and dying.

At some point, your friend may want to discuss his thoughts about dying. It can happen when you least expect it. Patients are often in a survival mode during treatment, sometimes focusing only on getting through the next hour. Then one day the doctor says: "The treatments are over, you are free to go. There's no sign of the cancer." As the patient enters remission, a flood of emotions may come raging forth. Dr. Gary Fleishman, a physician who was a member of Cancer Counseling's advisory board, once explained this onslaught of anxiety. "While patients are in treatment, they see us every day. There's always someone there for them, and we are actively fighting the disease. When that support is gone, it's very scary. It may be the first time they've allowed themselves to think about what might have happened or what could happen in the future." Although a patient may have looked death in the eye during treatment, it is only later that he is ready to talk about it.

Shelly, the woman who was concerned about both her parents when her father had cancer (see Chapter 1), was visiting him one afternoon. After three months of radiation treatment, his doctor told him he was cancer free. "You would think that would have been the happiest day of his life," recalls Shelly. "But he was depressed, miserable. Finally after much cajoling, he told me why. 'Shelly, I came that close to saying good-bye to this grand old life. I just never realized it until today. Now that the beast has had his way with me once, who is to say he won't come back? I just can't stop thinking about what would happen to your mama.'"

Fortunately, Shelly had been to a support group, so she didn't jump in and tell him not to think that way. She just listened as he reminisced about his life. He handed the living will over to her along with his legal information, then started talking about his funeral. "He wasn't morbid," Shelly said. "He just had to talk about it. What surprised me was that dying isn't such a horrible thing to discuss. Anticipating the conversation was worse than bringing it out in the open. He was a professor once, a proud and interesting man. For the first time in years, I saw that man again, the one I had always admired. Our discussion brought us closer than we had been in years. Perhaps because I was willing to listen, he was willing to share."

Over the years many people have told me they don't want to participate in a support group if any of the members are dying or are even going to discuss the subject. But being with someone who is dying, or has contemplated or faced death, is a privilege, one not to be taken lightly.

Lila let me spend hours at her home. A former group member, she could no longer leave her bed. On hot spring afternoons we would pass the time, she with her hands railing in the air, tossing them at some thought, some idea she was letting go of or pushing away. She was a brilliant and articulate woman. In those days together I learned my first real lessons about dying. It was as though she took my hand and showed me that part of my work. She died, so quietly, that although I was by her side, I did not see her leave. Walking beside her has improved my life in ways I cannot describe.

Of all the people who refused to sit in a room with a dying person, Carrie was probably the most afraid. However, she did join Lila's group. Carrie was the spokesperson at Lila's funeral. "I had never spoken to a group before," Carrie told me afterward, "let alone five hundred people. But I had to share the gifts that Lila bestowed upon me, and the only way I knew how to honor those lessons was by sharing them with the people who loved her."

If your friend or loved one wants to talk about dying, listen with an open heart. Don't cut him off or try to cheer him up. Just let him speak. Maybe you too will learn, as Shelly and Carrie did.

16. Look at illness as an opportunity to evaluate your life.

Coping with a life-threatening illness will inevitably trigger feelings about every other major loss you've experienced. Take this opportunity to review your past. Now is a good time to evaluate your expectations for the future and what life means to you.

Unfortunately, there's only one way through the pain, and that's through the pain. You cannot go around it or behind it or under it. You have to go through it.

Few people can pass through the cancer experience without evaluating, assessing, and learning something about their lives. You may learn something profound, or it may be something as simple as the importance of appreciating your surroundings. You may discover in concrete buildings a source of beauty and pleasure.

17. Forgive yourself, no matter how you react.

You won't say everything perfectly. You may also have feelings of anger and resentment that pop up and surprise you. Keep forgiving yourself.

Some Final Thoughts

Mitch, a patient we met in Chapter 1, describes how his fellow group members helped him deal with the cancer by following the guidelines presented in this chapter and the previous one. "It wasn't as much what they said as the fact that they stayed in constant contact with me and always offered support and followed through on whatever they offered to do," he says.

"I was especially grateful for the members who just listened. I probably told them the same things over and over, but they always appeared interested.

"I needed to talk about death and plans for my family. I didn't want to dwell on it, but I needed to plan and talk it through. It's like getting a flat tire. I don't think it will happen, but I carry a spare.

"I have children, and I wanted to find out how other people made living wills and financial plans. I really appreciated the members who would not only listen to my concerns but help me deal with these issues without judging me."

Stephanie, Mitch's wife, whom we also met in Chapter 1, got support from her childhood friends. These friends too had followed the guidelines in these two chapters. "They were always there for me," she says, "with their love and compassion. They also brought humor into my life. Some people just have that gift, and when they used it, it lit up my days. They didn't always take everything so seriously. They weren't intense all the time. They let me have moments when life wasn't serious. They helped me laugh at myself and the things I was going through. That's different from cheerleading. It's more from the heart, more genuine. It's not telling me, 'Cheer up. Everything will be fine.' It's not negating my feelings or concerns. It's knowing when to give me a break from the tough conversations."

Most of the families I have worked with over the years and those whom I interviewed for this book agree that the people who helped them the most were the ones that showed them love, nourished realistic hopes, and respected them.

In my twenty-three years of working in this field, I remember one comment in particular. "I don't really care what exact words people use to convey their feelings," Eliza said. "I don't expect my friends or relatives to be great orators, comedians, or therapists. All I want is for them to just call or visit once in a while and ask how I am. That's enough for me."

Some people need much more than Eliza. But most just want to know that you care and are there for them, and that on their journey, they are not alone.

And sometimes you won't be able to talk to them. Sometimes it's better to do other things to show you care. If you do talk to the person and you have shown him the kind of support Eliza describes, you can give to him in many other ways as well. The next chapter will help you generate ideas for gifts to give to patients and their loved ones.

Chapter 5

From the Goodness of Your Heart:
52 Gift Ideas

What Can I Do?

When someone we care about is ill, one of the first questions we ask is "What can I do?" This chapter will give you a list of 52 things you can do for patients and their families. If you are the primary caregiver, you may want to review this list. Highlight things your loved one needs, and the next time someone asks you, "What can I do?" you will have a clear idea about ways they can help.

If you are a friend, family member, or co-worker of the patient, there are so many things you can do. I hope this list will spark ideas to help you generate your own list. You may want to give copies of this book to others who want to help too. You can share these ideas with the family as well. Ask them to circle the items that they need or want. They can circle items they are interested in, and put stars by the ones they need most. Then make copies of the list and give them to their friends or family members.

When offering to help a family, be specific about how you can help. In Cancer Counseling's brochure *I Have Cancer, This Is What You Can Do,* Bob Davis writes, "One of the most hollow statements is, 'If I can be of help, call me.' While it is a nice gesture, it places the responsibility on me and my family to try to figure out what kind of help you are able to give, when you are willing to give it, how often, etc. . . .

"Think about the needs of the patient and the family. Then think about the kinds of things you can do best. This kind of thoughtfulness might lead you to the following kinds of expressions of support: 'You know I love yard work, and you may not be able to give that much attention now. I want you to forget it and leave it to me for a while.' 'I know you sometimes have to make a quick trip to the pharmacy. Next time call me, and I'll be happy to run that errand on a moment's notice.'"

Other statements you might say when you offer to help include:

> "You know I love to cook. You probably don't have time to cook now. I would like to fix your dinners for two weeks."
>
> "I'd love to come over every morning and make [the patient] breakfast while you get ready for work. Would that be helpful?"
>
> "I'm on my way to the supermarket. Is there anything I can get you?"
>
> "I'll be out at the mall on Saturday. Why don't you make a list of things you need, and I'll pick them up while I'm there."

Choose Wisely

Choose ways to help that fit your abilities. If you are the kind of driver who yells at anyone who gets in your way, don't offer to take the patient to doctors' visits. Jobs, gestures, and gifts ought to match your skills and interests.

Offer three specific choices. "I'm free on Saturday. I could run errands for you, pull weeds, or just come over and visit."

If you aren't sure how much time you have or how involved you want to get, offer to do one of the easier jobs on the list. Do not offer to visit if you aren't comfortable seeing the person or don't have time. Instead, send a card or call her. It's harder to cancel something that you have agreed to do than to add additional projects later.

Ask what the family needs first. You may think mowing the lawn would be helpful, but the husband may be planning to do that as a way to relax. You might assume everyone wants someone else to do their laundry. Some people prefer to do it themselves.

Most important, once you say you will help—do it. Keep your word, and be reliable. If you are not sure you can help, don't offer to. Wait until you have time. Most of the people I interviewed for this chapter made a point of saying that it wasn't the size of the gift that mattered. A handwritten note meant as much as or more than an elaborate gift.

Using the List

Some of the gifts listed here will be inappropriate at certain times. Others will never be appropriate in your situation. You have to decide which items fit your abilities and the family's needs.

The family may turn you down the first time you offer your assistance. Miranda, a college junior with leukemia, reflects on the offers friends made when she first became ill. "When I found out I was sick, I wanted to do everything myself. So I told everyone at school that I didn't need any help. I wish they'd ask to assist me now, because there are a lot of chores I can't do anymore."

One woman wanted to buy and decorate a Christmas tree the first year her husband was ill. She and her young boys enjoyed searching for the perfect tree. Three years later she had different priorities: "My sons were busy with school activities. Shopping for a tree by myself was a fiasco. I wanted to ask a neighbor to help, but I was afraid to impose."

If the family doesn't need your help now, wait a few weeks, then ask again. This month the husband may love taking care of his yard.

Three months from now, he may hate it. People may enjoy fixing meals at first, but later, they may welcome your ready-to-eat, home-cooked dinners.

Gestures

Many families need help with meals. When I asked two support groups, "What was the best gift anyone gave you?" every member answered, "Food." So this list starts with one of the easiest ways you can help—to give meals.

1. Bring food.
- Give ready-to-eat, complete meals.
- Pick up lunch on your way to visit, and set up a picnic by the person's bed.
- Send meals in microwave containers.
- Bring plates of goodies or boxes of crackers and cheese for the patient's other visitors.
- Schedule Meals on Wheels for people who qualify for this free service.
- Organize friends to take turns fixing dinners.
- Include sweets, health food snacks, or desserts for family members, especially children.
- Bring throw-away silverware and containers.
- Send baskets of fruit, bagels, or if you want to be extravagant, send a cold shrimp platter.
- Give gift certificates to restaurants that deliver.

2. Get the patient involved in activities that promote giving and improve his own self-worth.

Ask your friend or loved one to join you in church, charity, or school projects. Let him choose whether he wants to do something as rigorous as planning an event, or if he just wants to spend a few hours stuffing envelopes.

Patients and their family members who volunteered at my agency did everything from collecting items for silent auctions to writing newsletters to greeting guests at fund-raising events. They met others coping with cancer, developed friendships, and made contributions that made them feel good about themselves. They also learned new skills or realized they had had experiences they could use to help others.

If your friend does not want to get involved in one of these activities, perhaps you can teach her a new skill, such as how to sew or how to make something artistic. Then suggest you both donate your creations to a charity.

3. Send personal notes on a regular basis.

"I still remember the notes I received five years ago when I had cancer," recalled a patient.

A personal note does not have to be long. It can be anywhere from three lines to a few pages. Include pictures of your family. You can never send enough pictures of your kids to certain friends and relatives. Occasionally include a home video with your notes. A friend may not have an interest in your child's antics, but grandparents love them.

4. Help with chores related to seasons and holidays.

Put on snow tires. Plow the driveway. Take down the Christmas lights. Cover plants during storms. Rake leaves or take down screens or storm windows. A lot of these chores might otherwise go undone.

5. Help with out-of-town guests.

"I wanted to be at the hospital with my husband as much as I could. But when my parents stayed with me, they took hours to get ready to go see him. A neighbor offered to drive them to the hospital. She relieved a lot of the tension in my home," shares the wife of a patient.

Guests impose extra burdens on families. You can help out by transporting visitors, taking them out to dinner, providing a place for them to stay overnight, or making hotel arrangements.

6. Take and pick up laundry from cleaners.

7. Help around the house, or underwrite a cleaning service.

Before you do anything around someone's house, ask what they need done. If they cannot think of anything specific, then suggest chores you would like to do.

8. Call on a regular basis.

9. Visit.

One patient echoed the feelings of many when he said, "Some friends disappeared when I was going through treatment. A few of my co-workers visited every week for a few minutes. One lady came once a month. We talked for hours, and I always felt better after she left. It didn't matter how many times people came or how long they stayed—every visit was special."

Call first and ask the person: "Would you like company next week? When would be a good time for me to visit? I'll call before I come, just to make sure you're up to it."

10. Invite the person for a weekend getaway.

A two-day visit to a pretty area of your state can give a patient or a loved one a terrific break from doctors and hospitals and a stressful routine.

11. Continue to invite patients and caregivers to social functions, and be understanding of last-minute cancellations.

12. Help with pets.

"My wife hates cats. While I was in bed, my cat was sick. I was relieved when a friend took him to the vet for me."

"My husband travels a lot. My neighbors took turns walking our dog, bathing him, and buying his food."

Whether the family has fish, birds, turtles, or dogs, offer to help them take care of their pets.

13. Offer to be the point person—the scheduler.

A patient who thought her neighbors didn't care that she was in the hospital relayed this story: "I kept wondering why I didn't hear from Chet and Gwen. Then my sister told me they had been taking care of my garden."

Neighbors like Chet and Gwen aren't comfortable calling, but they may be giving in their own way. If you become the point person, you can let the family know about these special people. Work with the patient or the primary caregiver to organize support. Draw up a list of jobs they need done. Use this chapter to come up with ideas. Then solicit assistance from the friends who want to help. Keep a record of who is doing each job. Periodically, give the family a copy of the list with the names of the people who helped.

14. Offer to be the update person.

Ask the family if you can help them keep their friends and relatives informed about how the patient is doing. By updating others, you can save the family hours of repetitious phone calls. If you have a computer, you can send updates to friends and family members through the Internet.

15. Bring in the outside world with newspaper clippings and stories.

Share news about your office, neighborhood, family, or congregation. Talk about articles you have read in national newspapers. Bring pictures from an event.

16. Give catalogs.

Ask the family what types of items they need. Then arrange to have catalogs sent—to you, so the family doesn't throw them out with junk mail. This is especially helpful a few months before holidays, when patients are homebound or when caregivers are too busy to shop. Ask friends which catalogs they recommend.

The Innerbalance Catalog (800-345-3371) offers products like scented relaxation beads, a sunrise clock, and a white-noise machine. Levenger (800-544-0880) offers tools for serious readers, especially those who read in bed—including reading stands and reading pillows.

17. *Offer to baby-sit, organize weekends, or go shopping for children's needs—clothes, school supplies, or presents.*

18. *Invite the family over to share in a holiday celebration.*

19. *Offer to drive the children to their activities, like sports practice, doctors' appointments, or school functions.*

20. Make a date.

Invite the person to go with you to the zoo, to a museum, or to a play; to a matinee, dinner, or shopping spree; for a workout at your gym or for a walk in the neighborhood.

These kinds of dates meant a lot to one patient: "At first I made plans with friends, but I dreaded going. I was too tired or too busy. Eventually my attitude changed. These dates gave me something to look forward to. And I always felt better afterward."

A caregiver echoed a similar response. "I was so busy that I never made time for fun. When I finally accepted my friend's offer to go to the movies once a month, I immediately regretted it. This was crazy. I didn't have that kind of time for myself. Yet once I was there, I found it hard to think about my problems. Being away always revitalized me."

If she can't get away, offer to spend an afternoon with her sitting in the backyard or going for a drive, or ask her to show you her family album or old scrapbooks.

21. Create laughter in their lives.

- Memorize and tell a good joke.
- Tape or rent a comedy, and offer to bring it over with popcorn, pizza, or ice cream.
- Browse the comedy section of a bookstore, and buy a funny book or audiotape.
- Share funny memories of activities you did together.
- Ask if the patient would like you to bring your child with you when you visit. Kids have a wonderful way of making people laugh.
- Clip and send jokes from the Sunday comic strips.
- Tape-record a stand-up comic or one of the late-night talk shows.

22. Take the patient or the family to their favorite sporting event, or watch a game on TV together.

Buy tickets to the event, with the understanding that you may not stay for the whole game.

23. Help rent or pick up medical equipment.

24. Offer to buy and address holiday greeting cards.

25. Take the patient to get a wig or attend a class.

Patricia Semple of Elle Coiffures in Summit, New Jersey, recommends that you take the patient to a hair stylist before getting a wig. A stylist like Semple accompanies her clients herself when they go to pick out wigs. Then she takes them back to the hair salon and cuts their hair. The patient puts on the new wig, and then they both go out to lunch. "I encourage my clients to do this all in one day," says

Semple. "Otherwise it's too upsetting. I've been to many of these lunches. You should see how good my clients feel when a waitress or a stranger compliments them on their new hairstyle."

In partnership with the Cosmetic, Toiletry and Fragrance Association, the American Cancer Society provides a free program called Look Good...Feel Better. It helps patients cope with appearance changes by adapting hairstyles and makeup to their physical changes. These techniques can have a tremendous impact on self-confidence and ultimately on the whole recovery process. Offer to find out about this service and to drive the patient there. As Patricia Semple did, take her out after one of the lessons.

26. Offer to take notes during doctors' visits.

Even if the person tape-records visits, taking notes helps to organize the information better. If he doesn't have time to listen to the entire tape, notes can remind him of the parts he is interested in afterward.

27. Offer to do the family's holiday baking.

28. Help with shopping for birthdays, weddings, and special events.

Ask the family to make a list of the items they want for these special events, indicating price ranges. Even slightly dated catalogs can come in handy—family members can circle the gifts they want you to buy.

Offer to take them shopping if they are able to go with you. Ellen's friend Teddie stomped into Ellen's bedroom one day. "How about going with me on these shopping sprees?"

"But I can't even get out of bed," said Ellen. "I don't want to ride around in some old wheelchair."

"That's not what I had in mind," declared Teddie.

With Ellen curled up in the back of her minivan, Teddie would scavenge around, clutching Ellen's catalog pictures in her hands. They would go to smaller stores, ones they could park in front of, ones where Teddie could keep an eye on Ellen. Although she was too ill to get out of the minivan, Ellen soon came to enjoy these trips. Perched inside, she would read and gaze out the window, glad to even see a dump truck pass by, to see anyone going about the normal business of life. "Life does go on, and I'm still here, so I am going to enjoy what I can," said Ellen one day. "Hey, I'm enjoying just being out of bed."

And then there was Teddie's endearing routine. She would race out of the store, always announcing, while gasping for air, "I only have a second, I told the store manager the whole story, and he let me bring these out." Holding up her latest conquest, she'd say, "Well, which one do you like? Hurry up—the guy's going to be out here any minute!"

Ellen and Teddie have fond memories of those days, especially when they went shopping for Ellen's husband's birthday. Teddie raced out of stores, handing Ellen humorous, sexy, and sometimes disgusting cards, clothes, magazines, and tapes, ostensibly seeking her approval, "Hurry up, make up your mind—that manager is going to kill me!"

"Funny," Ellen said once her ordeal was over, "I'm all better now, but I miss those days. I would give anything to have just one of them again."

29. Leave notes in the car, in a briefcase, in a closet, or under a pillow.

Imagine you are driving to work, worried about the mother you have left sprawled across the bed. She looks sicker than you'd ever thought a human being could be. Then you open your briefcase, and a note falls out. You recognize your husband's handwriting. It is his latest joke of the month, or his urgent request for you to meet him for lunch in a hotel. Or maybe the note simply says, "I love you." Whether you leave such notes for the primary caregiver or the patient, they can be the little treats that keep them going.

30. Help organize financial papers or get insurance information.

These tasks are usually done by very close friends or family members, but even if you are not that close, you can still offer to help with these jobs. Maybe no one else has offered or wants to do them.

31. Make copies of all files, bills, and any other important records.

Copying is usually a job for someone very close to the patient—a family member, most often. However, if you have access to a copier and no one else does, you may be the perfect person to offer this service.

32. Offer to get the person's car washed or serviced.

Wash the car yourself, or hire a neighborhood child to do it. If your friend will allow you, take the car to get the tires or oil changed. Offer to provide rides to and from the service station or repair shop.

33. Buy an answering machine and teach the family how to use it.

Many elderly people have never considered using one of these. If you purchase one and show them how to use it, it can help them screen callers and avoid missing important calls.

Gifts

Besides doing things for patients and caregivers, you can also give them gifts. The gifts can be expensive or inexpensive, large or small. If you are not that close or if you are a co-worker, a large or expensive gift may be inappropriate. If your own family's large, you may want to all chip in and share the cost of a more expensive gift. The most extravagant gift that a client of mine received was a two-week cruise, which was given to her after she recovered from surgery. Her five children shared the expenses. The children enjoyed seeing their mother's happiness almost as much as she enjoyed the trip. The least expensive gifts, however, can sometimes be the most meaningful. One patient's children always managed to round up their own kids and include them in long and delightful phone conversations. You have to decide which gift best suits your friend or loved one.

1. Give books.

My clients have loved getting uplifting novels, mysteries, biographies, and the latest best-sellers. Give these books to patients and those close to them. Books that have inspirational or uplifting stories, like those compiled in *Chicken Soup for the Soul,* are great gifts for patients and caregivers.

Offer to pick up and return library books or tapes. Many libraries have services for the homebound and will mail out books free of charge to patients. Help the person set up this service. When he finishes reading a book, offer to return it for him. Mailing it back can be burdensome for a homebound patient.

2. Send humorous, entertaining, or inspirational magazines, newspapers, and cards.

"Mark your calendar with significant dates, such as annual checkups and birthdays," suggests Sister Alice Potts. "Then buy cards in advance, and save them in a file for those special times."

Ask the patient if he would like a subscription to *Coping,* to *USA Today,* or to a magazine related to his hobby.

3. Give a gift basket.

Include goodies such as a deck of cards or a special assortment of herbal teas, instant coffees, or wines.

4. Give a gift certificate to the family's favorite restaurant.

5. Give refundable or exchangeable tickets to the theater, opera, symphony, charity event, or comedy club.

6. Supply the patient with listening materials.

Chemotherapy and other treatments can affect one's ability to concentrate. Rent or buy books on tape or take out cassettes from your library.

7. Organize a resource notebook.

A notebook with a list of phone numbers and brochures from social service agencies and other resources will save the family hours of research. Use the Resources section of this book to gather the materials. The notebook can include where to get transportation, medical supplies, and counseling services.

Here's a sample page from a notebook:

Name of service
Phone number
Person you spoke with
What services they provide
When the services are available
Any comments or notes you have

Attach a brochure of the service.

8. Give or make something personal.

Pictures drawn by your children
A poem
A small framed painting
A quilt
A handmade sweater or shawl
Epsom salts or bubble bath in a decorated bottle
An heirloom

9. Give fun clothes or accessories—T-shirts, sweats, earrings, or jackets.

10. When the person is in the hospital, bring special treats.

Bring gifts for both patients and family members who are at the hospital. Items they might enjoy include a cooler with sodas, ice, bottled water, wine (with the hospital's permission), and snacks. A patient who has a longer stay might want exercise equipment, such as hand weights. Ask if the hospital will allow you to bring a stationary bike. Several bone marrow transplant patients I know have used these bikes during their long stays. Other gifts my clients have treasured are:

- A soft blanket
- A humorous coffee mug or large drinking cup
- A tiny photo album for a few special pictures
- A clock radio (specialty stores carry radios with sounds of waterfalls, rain, and the ocean)
- A comfortable decorated pillow
- An orthopedic foam wedge for the back (found at orthopedic supply stores)
- A pretty water pitcher
- A special head covering, such as a hat, visor, scarf, or baseball cap, or a cap with their favorite sports team's logo

11. Bring a gift that will encourage patients and primary caregivers to do something good for themselves.

Merry Templeton, an American Cancer Society volunteer, says that when she was hospitalized, the nicest gesture any of her friends made was to show up one day with bath oil and soaps. The woman offered to give Merry a sponge bath or shampoo, or to leave the gifts if Merry wanted to use them herself. Merry smiles when she remembers how great the bath made her feel.

Other gift ideas are:

A journal
A Day-Timer, to help them get organized

Nail, skin, and hair products
A gift certificate to a beauty salon
Relaxation tapes

Lucy Kim, the wife of a patient and a volunteer for Cancer Counseling, says that the most meaningful gift she got was nail polish. "It was my friend's way of telling me to take care of myself. It was the first time anyone gave *me* anything. More important, I had forgotten my femininity, wore raunchy clothes, didn't do my usual feminine things. The nail polish reminded me I was still a woman, and that made me feel so pampered."

12. Bring a board game, laptop computer, or card game.
Order the Klutz catalog (800-558-8944). Ask for item 4103, the *Classic Book of Board Games*, containing fifteen games, dice, and pieces for checkers. The games include backgammon, checkers, go, and fandango.

13. Pick up notepaper, and help with addressing or writing correspondence.

14. Buy bedside supplies.
You may not think these are important, but if you were confined to a bed or a hospital room, you would value them:

Post-It notes large enough to write lists on
Felt-tip or easy-to-press-down pens
Paper clips
A stapler
Tape
Spiral notepads
A mirror
Makeup organizer
Kleenex

Cotton balls
A calendar
Folders with pockets to keep brochures
Newspaper or magazine articles
Scissors

15. Give a sexy robe or special slippers.

Anything that makes a woman feel sexy or a man special will mean a lot. One woman told me, "I still treasure the sexy robe my husband gave me while I was in the hospital two years ago." Another woman cherishes the sexy nightgown that her female friends gave her.

Austin still traipses around the house in his favorite slippers—six years after his brother brought them to the hospital the night before a risky operation. "When my brother handed them to me and said, 'You'll be needing these,' it was his way of saying he believed I was going to survive."

16. Fill the room with flowers or blossoming plants.

- Bring or send flowers as often as once a week.
- Give fresh-cut flowers from your garden.
- Order an arrangement to be delivered to the hospital the night before surgery or the day someone returns home from the hospital. (Call the family to make sure flowers are allowed.)
- Give or send flowers as soon as you hear about the cancer. Include a personal brief note saying "I'm thinking about you," or "My prayers and thoughts are with you," or "I just want you to know how much I care about you."

17. Give a box of thank-you cards and a roll of stamps.

"Fifteen years ago," recalls Anne Root, a Cancer Counseling volunteer, "when I was recovering from surgery, a friend gave me a roll of postage stamps and a box of cards. These can be the hardest items to find when you are in the hospital."

18. Send a gift certificate for a four-hour limousine ride, a massage, or a weekend getaway at a cozy hotel.

If your loved one or friend likes spontaneous events, a limousine can be a great treat. Imagine her walking out her front door to find a limo waiting to escort her around the city or to her favorite restaurant.

Or perhaps your friend would just like a weekend to herself or with her husband. A gift certificate to a cozy hotel may be just the encouragement she needs to make plans.

19. Give a donation to a charity in the person's name.

However you choose to show you care, your friend or loved one is going to appreciate it. Although some of the gifts I have listed are elaborate and expensive, any gift you give from the heart is priceless. Fifteen years after her hospitalization, Anne Root remembers the friend who gave her a roll of stamps—not because of the size of the gift itself but because the person who gave it cared about her.

Again, many of these gifts are appropriate not only for patients but for their caregivers as well. Family members and loved ones need your love, your gifts, your surprise treats, and your gestures of kindness as much as, and in some ways more than, the patient does. Too often, the family members are neglected while the world revolves around the patient. Too often, loved ones experience isolation and depression. But you can change that, not only by giving a gift but by providing the support and assistance they need. The next chapter will teach you how to help and comfort the person closest to the patient, the primary caregiver.

Chapter 6

The One Who Needs You: Providing Comfort to the Primary Caregiver

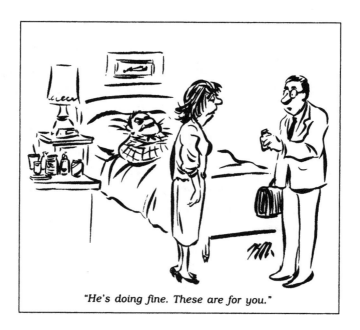

"He's doing fine. These are for you."

Mary Dee Neal, a board member of the Ballet Guild International, told me that she "became a caregiver right in the middle of making a plan to adopt a child. Now finally, six years later, I'm able to carry on with that plan. I learned a lot in the intervening years. And I'm here to say that you can't change what happens, but you can control your attitude." For Mary Dee, as for many caregivers, it all happened very quickly. Within eighteen months she became a caregiver not only to her mother but to her brother and her mother-in-law. She and I met when her brother was in the hospital. At that time there were problems with his wife, his doctors, and his treatment. Mary Dee was smart—she didn't try to take all these problems on herself. She reached out to Cancer Counseling for moral support, advice, and guidance.

One important thing she did was to take care of herself. She kept her career, her husband, and her friends all in balance. She had to—it was the only way she could help anyone. But what really got her through her years of caregiving was her friends. They understood that she needed their love and compassion, and they found ways to give it, sending humorous cards, notes, and flowers.

Her friends' support enabled Mary Dee to help all those who needed her. "What I remember most was this one friend," she says, "who came by my house when I wasn't home. She handed my houseguest a bottle of champagne, in a gorgeous bucket with two glasses inside. A note was attached, saying simply, 'Cheers.' When I saw it on the kitchen counter, it made me laugh, I felt so wonderful. I felt pampered because it was such a wonderful luxury. I knew she really cared about me. And that's what made all the difference over those years—friends like her.

"Today there's a child out there who doesn't have a parent. And now my husband and I can go back to those other plans, finding and adopting that child."

After you read this chapter, think of Mary Dee and the child waiting for her. If anything had happened to her, if she had not gotten the support she needed, she might not have had the energy to fulfill that dream. Think of that child who will be fortunate enough to find a home. The love you give to a primary caregiver can affect the patient as well, not to mention hundreds of others in ways you might not even imagine. As I started this story, I mentioned that Mary Dee is with the ballet. I left out that she is providing a home for a local dancer who cannot afford one. She and her husband raise thousands of dollars to help charities (including mine). She has given back the love that her friends gave her to so many others. So you see, whether you give champagne or a card or follow any of the suggestions in this book, you can make a major contribution not only to the caregiver but to hundreds of people you may never know.

A chronic or life-threatening illness places a tremendous burden upon those closest to the patient. In addition to taking on many responsibilities, loved ones experience the heart-wrenching pain of helplessly watching someone they love suffer.

In my support groups I have discovered that both male and female caregivers exhibit symptoms of psychological and physiological stress, including the exacerbation of preexisting illnesses, migraines, depression, and digestive and sleeping disorders.

In my couples' groups, I found that both those who had successful relationships and those who had serious marital differences had emotional problems associated with the cancer. A bad marriage did not insulate couples from experiencing psychological pain.

I found similar problems in my family support groups. Family members who have taken on primary caregiving responsibilities often say that taking care of a loved one is a draining and usually an overwhelming twenty-four-hour-a-day career. It can lead to a host of secondary stress-related problems.

Dr. Ken Kopel, a former president of the Houston Psychological Association, gives this perspective on spouses as caregivers:

"I've seen countless couples who don't talk about the most important issues that are going on with them. As a result, the spouse who is the caregiver has to handle the pain by herself. She has to put on the fake happy face. She walks around ready to explode. And in so doing, she goes through a tremendous number of emotions.

"One of the most powerful feelings is guilt: 'Did I do enough?' I come across women trying to be nurse, wage-earner, mother, wife, and friend, doing it all, to the point they are busy twenty hours a day. They are exhausted, and yet they tell me, 'I don't know if I have done enough.' They think this is their last chance to do something. If the final moment comes and they haven't done all they can, they have to live with it the rest of their lives."

Besides guilt and concerns about doing enough, Dr. Kopel adds, "those feelings get caught up with, 'I don't want to do this, but the patient wants me to. I'm going to do it even though it's against my better judgment.'"

He continues, "There are all kinds of intricate reasons why this goes on, and it's not always because they have a deep profound love for their spouses. Their own issues may be driving them." Perhaps their mother acted this way, and she is the only role model they have.

Another underlying factor driving these caregivers is their fear of losing their loved ones. The death of a spouse is one of the most stressful events an individual can experience. Anticipating this loss, living with the possibility every day, is stressful as well. And when a parent is ill, an adult child faces losing his history, a part of his identity, and in some cases his best friend.

To live with this disease is to live with uncertainty and ambiguity. Even when the patient is cancer free, caregivers live with the fear that it may return.

Dr. Kopel describes other reactions that primary caregivers have. "They feel angry and helpless at having to do things they never wanted to do—write the checks, keep the books, drive the kids to school, manage the car repairs, clean the house, shop for the children's clothes and schedule their appointments. They overreact and get angry when hospital workers take too much time bringing food or medicine. They lash out at anything that is concrete to release their emotions."

Coping Styles

Typically, families deal with an illness the way they have dealt with other problems. If their style is to argue, they will continue to argue. If they normally withhold their feelings, they will remain silent. Some families pull together, resolving smaller problems so that they can meet the larger ones. In other families, underlying issues rise to the surface, and their ability to handle them may well be impaired. Preexisting conflicts become more severe. Unfortunately, the familiar coping methods that have served them well may no longer suffice.

What You Can Do

You aren't going to solve all the caregiver's problems. You shouldn't even try. But you can show her different ways to cope. You can bring joy into her life, as Mary Dee's friends did. You can provide assistance that lightens her burden. You can try to understand the situation from her perspective. You can share insights that give her hope, and humor that brings her laughter. You can point out alternatives that may never have occurred to her. You can show her a road she might never have known was there. These are all ways you can be helpful to the caregiver. But the only way to know for sure you are helping is to ask the person what she needs.

The suggestions in Chapters 3 and 4 are the foundation for the guidelines in this chapter. But the most important guideline is: *Ask first*. Ask the primary caregiver what she needs from you and how you can help. Listen to her response—it may surprise you.

Jeffrey spent thousands of dollars and many hours commuting home to help his parents on the weekends when his mother was undergoing radiation. Exhausted, he dragged himself into one of my support groups. "They need me," he said. "They can't take care of themselves."

He described what it was like at his parents' house: "My dad works long hours, and Mom is at the hospital for treatment all week. They have this rambling old home with endless rooms, and a huge yard that needs to be maintained. I take care of the yard and help with the house on the weekends because Dad can't."

I said, "But the weekends may be the only time they have to themselves. Have you asked your parents whether they need you every weekend?"

"I never thought of asking them."

During the next visit Jeffrey asked his parents how often they really needed his help. They were always happy to see him, they replied. But if he visited only once a month and called more frequently, he would be giving them the kind of support they needed. In other words, they wanted his assistance, but not as often as he had assumed they did.

The following guidelines suggest specific ways you can help the primary caregiver in your life.

1. Help him focus on his own well-being.

Dr. Alan Valentine, a psychiatrist at M. D. Anderson Cancer Center, suggests asking the caregiver about his basic needs: "Are you eating well, exercising, and sleeping?"

Try to ask without being oversolicitous. If you push too hard, admonishing her to take care of herself, she may be offended or simply ignore you.

2. Don't let the patient be the focus of all of your conversations.

Peggy stormed into one of my support groups bursting at the seams. Frustrated, she sank into a chair, and releasing a long sigh, she said, "I can't walk down the hall at work or shop at the market without someone asking me, 'How's Ryan?' You may think I'm ungrateful. At least everyone cares enough to ask how his treatments are going. I appreciate the concern, but after seven months, I'm tired of answering the questions. And when I'm out at the store, it's the only time I have to myself."

A few weeks later, she strolled into group, exuding her first smile in months: "I was in the same fancy new supermarket I go to every Saturday. I was ready. I had my polite face on, and I was going to be positive about the Ryan questions. Then Wendy, a woman whom I barely know, approached me. She had that look, that curious I-can't-wait-to-ask-about-that-poor-sick-young-husband-of-yours look. She appeared so concerned, I was worried she wanted to pray right there in the aisle or ask me to recite a dissertation on our most *regrettable* circumstances. Instead, this gentle lady took my arm and whispered, 'This probably isn't my place, dear, because we aren't that close, but lately I've been worried about you. How are you handling all this?'

"I was caught off guard and so touched that I started to cry right there, in the aisle, leaning over my cat food, paper towels, and macaroni. All this woman did was ask me how I was doing. I was so drained, I didn't even know how to answer. Then she asked if I had a few minutes to sit down for a cappuccino. Uh-oh, I thought, she's just like all the rest. She's going to grill me about Ryan.

"For some reason, I agreed anyway. We wheeled our carts over to a café in the store and settled into a plastic-flowered booth in a very private corner. And I ended up talking for what seemed like hours."

Three months later, Wendy was one of Peggy's closest confidantes. They met once a week and shared a cup of coffee. Although they talked about Ryan, he was never the main focus of their conversations.

3. Encourage time outs and baby steps.

Nita, a woman in her sixties, wanted time for herself, away from her husband, Chuck, who was in his sixth month of chemotherapy treatments. Yet she felt guilty about wanting it. "Chuck whines and sometimes yells if I'm gone for even an hour," she complained to a friend. The friend encouraged Nita to join one of my support groups.

After a few weeks Nita told the group, "This place is my only break. It means so much to me to come here every week. Now I want more time away on my own—time to get my hair done or browse through one of those huge bookstores."

The group offered to provide sitter services for three hours on Wednesdays. They would take turns keeping Chuck company. It was difficult for Nita to accept their offer, but it was even harder for her to tell Chuck she needed more time by herself.

She had taken the first step, but not for several months was she comfortable about taking the second. Eventually she agreed to schedule two hours each Wednesday for "mall walking," bookstore browsing and lunch with friends. The group would look after Chuck.

This fixed schedule also helped Chuck know what to expect each week. Although he still objected occasionally, Nita knew that if she was going to be the best caregiver she could, she had to take care of herself too. She also realized it was good for him to have other people to depend on.

By attending the Monday group and her Wednesday "time outs," she was able to venture into this new schedule at her pace. Once she was comfortable about being away, she was willing to set aside even more time for herself.

4. Respect private spaces and the need for solitude.

Elena had always admired her parents' relationship. Married for fifty-two years, they were inseparable and affectionate, and they respected each other. Now she learned that her mother was hospitalized and would undergo surgery. Rushing to her mother's hospital bedside, Elena arrived just as the rising sun was piercing through the windows. Her father, who had obviously shared the narrow metal bed with her mother the night before, was shaving. "Where's Mom?" Elena whispered. Her father tilted his head toward the closed bathroom door. "She's getting ready. They'll be here any minute. The surgery is in an hour."

Elena plopped down onto her mother's bed. "How are you holding up, Father?"

Always one to be cordial to his children, but reveal little, he turned to her with reddened eyes and said, "I'm doing my best."

Elena felt helpless. It would be her mother's third operation, yet she still didn't know how to ask her father how he was doing, even though the stress was obviously tearing him apart.

Her mother emerged from the tiny bathroom. "I'll be okay. Don't look so worried, you two." Before Elena could reply, an orderly appeared at the door, and her mother was whisked away.

Seven hours later, a nurse strode into the waiting room, clasping surgical reports. Elena's father, worn out from nights of worrying, was ecstatic when the nurse told him that the doctors were closing up his wife and the cancer had not spread. Elena assumed he'd want to celebrate or, at the very least, have lunch with her. Instead, he said he wanted to go home and be by himself.

Elena hesitated, wanting desperately to stay with him. Then she rubbed his shoulders and told him to go ahead. "I knew he was grateful for my company, and as much as I wanted to be with him, I realized he just needed to be alone."

It may be especially hard to give someone space if you've traveled a long way to help him, as Elena had. Your loved one is undoubtedly grateful for your support, but he still may need time alone to regroup, to replenish his strength, and to fortify himself for the challenges that lie ahead.

5. Help prevent burnout.

Let's say you have a supercaregiver on your hands—someone approaching burnout, as Dr. Kopel described, someone busy twenty hours a day. There are people who can handle this pace, but your supercaregiver looks awful, and she's lashing out at anyone and everyone who crosses her path. She's alienated her friends, kicked out her beloved cat, and ignored her kids, and her car has had a few accidents, for which she claims she was not to blame. What do you do?

Social worker Diane Blum, the director of Cancer Care, recommends that you "try and describe some of the behavior" to the caregiver herself. "Say, 'This is a very difficult time, and I want you to know I'm concerned, but it seems to me that you're not yourself.' Another way to approach the person is to say, 'In my experience, many people who are in your situation feel stressed.' This allows the caregiver to say, 'Me too.' It takes the stigma out of her feelings."

Dr. Alan Valentine acknowledges how difficult it is to support supercaregivers in taking care of themselves. "Sometimes it's hard to save them from themselves," he says. "You have to respect that they want to do what they are doing. It's what works for them."

Caregivers may appear overworked, but for some of them, this is their method for coping. They function better if they are busy.

However, if you notice that the caregiver who concerns you is drinking too much or abusing drugs, Diane Blum suggests you bring in a professional who is trained to do interventions.

The following signs of distress should also alert you to encourage the caregiver to seek professional counseling:

Withdrawal from friends and family
Pathological guilt ("It's my fault he has cancer.")
Suicidal feelings ("I don't deserve to live.")
Severe depression ("I feel worthless." "I can't stop crying.")
Sleeping or eating disorders
A significant change in weight

6. Don't be a backseat driver.

Sometimes caregivers are additionally burdened by interfering relatives. "My mother-in-law constantly points out that I'm not doing enough for Marie or my three boys," says David. "First of all, my mother-in-law doesn't live with us. How can she possibly know what I do? Criticizing me only causes more tension.

"There are days I come home thinking, I can do this, I can handle this. Then my mother-in-law calls. By the time I get off the phone, I feel defeated and upset.

"She's always giving me advice: 'I know Marie better than you, and you should...' 'You shouldn't work such long hours.' 'You should be more concerned about...' 'You act like you're waiting for her to die when you treat her like this.'

"I realize my mother-in-law feels out of control. She probably thinks she's helping by offering me her opinions. But her advice and badgering only make this harder on my boys, myself, and Marie."

David's overbearing mother-in-law may be an extreme example. You may make similar comments even though you didn't mean to interfere.

You may think you know the patient better than the caregiver does, or that you can improve the patient's care. You may be right. Yet the primary caregiver may be offended if you try to intervene the way Cynthia did.

"I had a screaming fight with my seventy-year-old aunt," says Cynthia. "I'm a nurse, and I knew my uncle wasn't taking care of himself. I even offered to arrange to take him back to his oncologist. But she hit the ceiling. 'How do you know what's best for us? Just because you're a nurse, you're still only in your twenties! How dare you tell us how to handle this!' "

Other comments that caregivers hate include:

> "I know the patient is going to be fine, if you..."
> "When are you going to..."
> "Don't you think you should..."
> "You shouldn't leave her with help. What if something happens?"
> "Can't you find someone else to do that?"

If the primary caregiver has solicited your support, give it. However, if you make recommendations when she has not asked for your help, you appear to be a backseat driver. You have not been invited into the car, yet you want to tell them how to drive it.

You are walking a fine line. Although you may have more expertise or skills than the primary caregiver, you have to be careful not to alienate her. Of course, if you think she is being neglectful and causing harm or pain to the patient, consult with a doctor or professional therapist about how best to approach the caregiver.

7. Keep the relationship two-sided.

As we have seen, Peggy had difficulties with her friends while she was caring for her husband, Ryan. "I hated it when my friends and co-workers stopped talking about the things we had talked about before Ryan was sick. I still wanted people to lean on me when they were having problems," she explained. "I didn't want to monopolize the relationships, and it felt awful when they stopped asking me for advice. It was as if they were either protecting me, or they assumed I was interested only in Ryan."

This does not mean you have an open invitation to complain to a friend who has become a caregiver. You have to be aware if he appears to be overloaded and unable to listen to one more problem. Nevertheless, if you asked him for advice and shared mutual interests with him before his wife got cancer, you need to continue to do so.

Peggy still wants her friends to need her. Being needed and being able to support others makes her feel good about herself and worthwhile.

If you bring up a problem, however, and she doesn't show any interest, change the subject. Save it for another time.

8. Offer only help that you can and are willing to give.

Imagine trying to care for a patient as well as completing an endless list of household and family chores. One day your neighbor Alex visits and offers to help you. You're relieved. You think, "I'm not alone. I don't have to do it all. Maybe I will even get an extra hour to myself." Alex says, "I want to take your kids to the zoo with me on Wednesday."

Wednesday arrives. You're at the hospital with your husband, and you call home to check your messages. When you hear Alex's voice, dread travels down your spine. Then he apologizes. He can't pick up your kids today. "Maybe next week," he says.

You're forty-five minutes away. Your husband is in a closed-off room undergoing radiation. You can't tell him the kids have to be picked up. You yell at the nurses as you race out the door. At that moment you wish you had never met Alex.

Another example: Your neighbor Celia tells you, "I'll bring dinner over next Tuesday." On Tuesday you work a few extra hours at the office, explaining to your kids and husband that Celia will provide dinner. "Don't worry, it's all taken care of," you say.

It's Tuesday at seven o'clock. You stroll in from your first productive workday in months. You actually sang along with the radio on the way home. You feel good for the first time in weeks. A now-very-hungry-and-agitated family greets you at the door, wearing a how-could-you-do-this-to-us expression? Your refrigerator is empty. Celia calls. "I'm sorry I forgot to pick up dinner. Can I do it next week?" It doesn't seem like much, but to a family in turmoil, such a cancellation may seem like a last straw.

Emergencies happen, and once in a while you may not be able to keep a plan or give the help you've offered. At the very least notify the family as soon as you can. Then try to find someone else to fill in.

If you have shared carpools with other parents and you cannot make your turn, take the initiative to replace yourself if you have to cancel. If you were bringing a meal and you know that four other people assist with meals, see whom you can switch with. If no one can help, call and have something delivered.

Don't offer to do a service when you know in advance that you are going to be stretched for time. Do your best to make plans only when you think you can keep them.

And when you offer support, be specific. Say, "I would like to give you a break. Tell me when I can take you to dinner or for coffee in the next two weeks." Or: "I have time on Fridays and Sundays—would you like me to come over and keep the patient company so you can have some time for yourself?"

Remember, one of the hardest things caregivers experience is asking others for help. Some are overwhelmed and don't know what they need. Others are uncomfortable about asking or are so busy, they think that stopping long enough to figure out what others can do would take more effort than just doing it themselves. If you make it easier for a caregiver to ask you for help, she may be more willing to relinquish some of her responsibilities, not only now, but in the future.

9. Give plenty of hugs.

Cancer is a family illness. The patient's loved ones are hurting too. They need your affection and understanding as much as the patient does.

Friends and other visitors often neglect the needs of the caregiver. Sometimes they'll comfort children but not the person closest to the patient. When they enter the home, they focus only on the patient's needs.

A few hugs, a smile, a pat on the shoulder—any show of affection can make an enormous difference to a caregiver. There are days they may need your hugs more than the patient does.

Jody described what hugs meant to her as the wife of a patient: "I was exhausted from working nineteen hours a day and being everything to everyone—Trey, the children, his parents, his friends. When people would visit, they'd ask me to cater to them. Could I get this one little thing for them? They never thanked me. They brushed past me when they came in, and they'd leave without saying good-bye. There were days I hurt so badly, and no one noticed.

"Then Trey's sister would visit. When she walked in our home, she always came up and hugged me. It was the only time I felt like someone understood what I was going through. Next she'd round up the kids and hug them too. Trey and I both appreciated her affection more than any words she could have said."

10. Compliment the caregiver on a difficult job well done.

Leon's wife, Charlene, had a tougher time with each subsequent round of her chemotherapy. Leon spent as much time with her as he could. He also took care of the children and the household and maintained a demanding career.

When the holidays rolled around one year, he climbed up a ladder to decorate the front door with a string of white lights. Shanna, the next-door neighbor and Charlene's best friend, had long admired the way Leon supported his wife. When Charlene noticed him on the ladder, she bundled up and went over to see if she could help.

"No, thanks," he said. "I like doing this."

Then Shanna realized how little he complained about all of his responsibilities and how hard he worked to keep joy in Charlene's world. Looking up at Leon, she said, "I've never told you this, but I just want to thank you for all you've done for my best friend. You've been so good to her."

Leon scrambled down the ladder. "You think so?"

Shanna nodded. "Charlene's always talking about how kind you are to her and the kids."

Leon shuffled his feet. Staring at the ground, he replied, "You know, no one's ever told me that except Charlene. It means a lot to me that someone else has noticed."

11. Even when you don't get along with the primary caregiver, try to be polite.

"I detest my stepfather. He's a mooching, lazy, loud, obnoxious pest. I hate the way he takes care of Mom, and I'd like to just kick him out of their house. Of course I can't do that," says Sheila, the daughter of a patient.

"The least he could do is stop answering the phone. I have to go through him every time I want to speak to her. I know he savors being her gatekeeper and picking fights with anyone who calls her. He never fails to bring up some topic that he knows infuriates me. By the time I talk to her, I'm a mess."

You don't have to let yourself be bullied by a gatekeeper like Sheila's stepfather, but you do have to find a way to get along. He may be the last person you feel like supporting, but aggravating him or confronting him will serve only to upset you and eventually the patient.

Imagine what Sheila's stepfather does after he hangs up the phone. He stomps into his wife's room and yells, "I can't stand that kid of yours." Or he whines, "Why does your daughter have to be so rude to me?" The wife, already well aware of the conflict, is now confronted with a problem she can't solve and doesn't need to be part of. Even if the stepfather never mentions Sheila to her, the friction is present.

When you call, be polite. Keep it short.

If you had a boss you couldn't stand but you needed the job, you'd find a way to appease him. You don't have to become the caregiver's best friend. In spite of your animosity, you can try to be understanding, even inquisitive. Once in a while you could ask the caregiver how he is holding up. You can stop even the rudest person dead in his tracks, if you treat him with concern and compassion.

12. Help with children.

Offer to keep the patient company so that her husband can spend more time with his kids, or take their kids out for something fun. You can also help kids with homework, hobbies, or sports. Think of ways to include their children in your own activities. Children often feel neglected when their parents are ill because they are no longer the first priority. By giving this kind of help, you are doing two things: easing the child's worries about being rejected and helping parents with child care.

13. Provide hospital breaks.

Many patients need to be surrounded by family or friends while they are in the hospital. And I've seen hundreds of spouses who will rarely leave patients' rooms. Yet when a friend offers to sit with the patient for a while, the caregiver will usually agree to take a break. She'll take time for herself even if she doesn't leave the hospital grounds, by going for walks or visiting the gift shop, library, or chapel.

The Caregiver Needs You as Much as the Patient Does

Couples in my support groups often referred to the cancer as "our" disease. In many ways this illness belongs to the caregiver as much as it does to the patient. Many patients have told me that the disease was harder emotionally on their loved ones than on themselves.

Cancer can permeate every area of a caregiver's life. Your kind words or acts of kindness will brighten her day and ease her load. And maybe you can help her take care of herself while she is caring for the patient. As a friend or relative, you will have many opportunities to help. Even if you live far away, you can always call, always be a sounding board, a warm voice, the comforting presence of someone who cares.

There are also opportunities to support caregivers in the workplace. The next chapter will show you how to help a co-worker who is either a caregiver or a patient.

Chapter 7

Managing Cancer in the Workplace: Taking Care of Employees While Meeting Your Goals

Dean was a gregarious, successful sales representative. He liked his job and was good at it, until a tiny cancerous lump invaded his career, his home, and every aspect of his life. As three months of radiation loomed ahead of him, he knew his work was going to suffer. Still, determined to do the best job he could, he scheduled his therapy for Fridays and continued to be productive Tuesdays through Thursdays. His manager, Carey, agreed to this schedule and accommodated Dean whenever he needed additional time off.

That was seven years ago. Dean is now a regional sales manager. He attributes a good part of his success to Carey, who is now a vice-president. Other companies have offered Dean jobs, but he remains loyal to his boss: "I want to stay with the company and the people who treated me with dignity and respect during the toughest days of my life. Carey gave me the opportunity to do my job, which I could still do well, although I felt helpless in every other area of my life. I'll always believe he had something to do with why I'm alive today."

Companies manage employees coping with cancer in a variety of ways. Whether it is the employee who has the disease or a family member, it can significantly affect the person's productivity or, in the case of a small company, the very survival of the organization.

When an employee is ill, co-workers usually experience feelings of shock, denial, and fear—fear that it could happen to them; fear that they won't know what to say or do; and fear of losing part of their team. An ailing co-worker can also remind colleagues of problems and feelings they would rather not think about at the office.

Because cancer arouses these fears, some patients and their loved ones receive unsupportive behavior from co-workers. So they may initially decide not to disclose information about the disease. Despite their silence, the fact they are living with the disease will usually surface when performance declines or if a co-worker finds out about it. In some cases, fellow team members may become aware of the problem but contribute to the denial because they don't know how to address a catastrophic illness in the workplace.

Employers often have misconceptions about cancer based on personal experiences that have no parallel with the actual issues this particular employee is facing. I've heard employers make comments such as, "When my father had cancer, he couldn't work, so this employee must not be able to work either." And: "When my sister had cancer, she wanted to use her job as an escape. So my employee must want to keep all of her responsibilities for the same reason."

Regardless of such preexisting fears and attitudes, co-workers and employers can develop considerate approaches when an employee becomes a patient or a primary caregiver. The following guidelines may be adapted to fit your own office situation. They are equally applicable when you are working with employees with cancer or employees who are caregivers.

Guidelines for the Owner, Manager, or Supervisor

Don't participate in denial. Talk about health-related issues as soon as you become aware of them.

What plans does the employee have? What benefits will he need? What kind of schedule and workload will he be able to handle? Discuss the situation with him to determine what he is able and unable to do.

Your company may offer services that he is unaware of. Give him the name and phone number of the employee benefits office manager. Make sure he has up-to-date copies of company brochures about insurance benefits and support services. He may have received these when he was hired, but he will need current information, including phone numbers.

Arrange to accommodate the employee in any way you can. Your actions will demonstrate your compassion and set an example for others as well. If you ignore an employee who you know is battling the disease, six months later you may have to deal with his depression, alcoholism, or poor performance.

Don't reduce the employee's responsibilities without discussing them with him.

Patients and their loved ones suffer many blows, and reduced job responsibilities is one of them. It conveys yet another negative message and fuels the most common fears: fear of losing a part of their identities, their jobs, health insurance, and income.

Ask the employee to participate in delegating his responsibilities, if that becomes necessary.

Before Gina, a well-respected employee, underwent radiation, she told Marshall, her supervisor, that she couldn't maintain her workload for the next two months.

He asked her what areas of her job she wanted to delegate. After they talked, he called a staff meeting to inform her co-workers.

Gina said later, "I really respected him for helping me maintain my job. He had allowed me to focus on the work I could do well and to decide which tasks I wanted to delegate."

Meet with the entire team to delegate the workload.

During the staff meeting, Marshall explained to the team the agreements that Gina and he had made. The co-workers were more than willing to pitch in and help with the tasks Gina had relinquished.

If Marshall had made the decision without consulting Gina, the others might have resented the extra workload, or Marshall, or even Gina.

Conducting a group meeting made it easier for Marshall to distribute the workload than meeting with employees individually would have done. Meeting together gave the co-workers a sense of ownership and accountability toward their added responsibilities.

A word of caution: Some people do want their workloads reduced, as Gina did. Others want them to remain the same. As a supervisor, you will have to make the ultimate decision about whether to reduce responsibilities. Your decision can affect the entire company.

Morgan was having a problem with a co-worker at his office. "Melanie and I are managers in an accounting firm," he told me. "We've been pretty close since we started here. She's never hesitated to tell me about her love life, her family, or her cancer. We've talked openly about it from the beginning.

"She's had to leave the office early every day for her radiation therapy. I know she's taken extra files home so as not to affect her productivity. She told me she *assumed* her supervisor would be satisfied with this schedule change. She seemed to handle her workload without any problems. But then Melanie withdrew from me, stopped confiding in me. Around the same time, the rest of us were assigned some of her clients. I thought she had initiated the transfers, so I didn't mention them to her. I did wonder why she stopped talking to me. Occasionally, I'd ask about her treatments, but her answers were abrupt. So I stopped asking, respecting her privacy. I figured she just wanted to focus on work and that our old relationship would resume when the treatments ended.

"Now she seems depressed. She's rude to her staff. She's barely talking to anyone here. We're worried about her, but we don't know what to do. And I'm not sure if she's upset about the cancer or losing her clients. How can I support her without prying? Apparently she no longer wants to talk to me."

I encouraged Morgan to have Melanie call me. As it turned out, she was doing quite well with her treatments and was pleased they were almost over. But she wasn't pleased with her supervisor for transferring her clients, or with her co-workers for accepting them. "I didn't say anything when the boss took my accounts away," she told me. "He never asked me what I wanted, and I didn't confront him. I depended on my work to keep me focused on something positive. Now I don't even feel useful there."

With her permission, I explained her feelings to her supervisor. He replied in surprise, "I thought I was doing Melanie a favor. I don't know what her problem is. I wanted to help, so I reduced her workload by reassigning some of her clients to her colleagues." Not only had his actions hurt Melanie, they had disrupted the entire office.

Grady, a manager from a large paper company, sums up the problem that employers face: "It's difficult to decide what is a fair balance for the employee, what will let him keep his job and financial status while maintaining his self-image.

"I've found that the best way to handle this is to talk openly and honestly with the employee about what I expect from him. I include him in making any decision that affects his job. I reevaluate whatever responsibilities he has on a regular basis, even weekly if necessary."

Be flexible about schedules.

Although some companies now have flextime, many do not. Be willing to alter the work schedule of someone living with a catastrophic illness.

By being flexible with her hours, you will reduce some of the burdens she would be under if she had to maintain a rigid schedule.

Whether you've changed her hours or her responsibilities, reevaluate the arrangement on a regular basis, weekly or biweekly. Adjust schedules and jobs as circumstances change.

WHEN WORK IS DISRUPTED, A LOT MORE THAN THE JOB IS COMPROMISED

Watch for signs of trouble.

Anxiety, depression, withdrawal, tardiness, poor performance, and abrupt or rude behavior toward other employees are signals that the employee is in trouble. Slamming down the phone, yelling at inanimate objects, and banging doors may be normal behavior for some people. However, if you know the person is dealing with cancer, talk about the situation before it escalates. Show compassion toward him while clearly stating the problems his behavior is causing.

If the employee's behavior is disrupting the workplace, you as the supervisor will have to confront the issue. He may insist that his loved one's illness or his own isn't upsetting him. Yet when he is irritable or not performing his job, social worker Diane Blum, the executive director of Cancer Care, suggests that you "try to describe some of the behaviors. Say, 'This is a very difficult time, and I want you to know I'm concerned. It seems to me that you're not yourself. Please let me know how I can help.' Or you can say, 'In my experience, many people in your situation feel like they can't cope.'

"By letting the employee know you understand how stressful this is, you take away the stigma for him of admitting he has a problem. It allows him to respond, 'That's how I feel.' "

Next, clearly identify the specific behavior you want changed without attacking the employee himself. For example, you could say, "I want to support you, but I'm having a problem with your reports coming in so late. Is there a way we can resolve this problem together?" Or: "I know you are having a tough time, and I'm very sorry. But we have to find a way to work it out without yelling at the staff. They care about you and it's hard for them to deal with the anger."

Be willing to assign temporary jobs on an ongoing basis.

At times you may have to reduce the employee's workload. You may need a task to be completed, and you can't be flexible. Or she may be jeopardizing the safety or productivity of others. When circumstances like these arise, try to give her a temporary assignment. Let her return to her original assignment when you have both decided she is ready.

The Resources section of this book lists other sources of referrals to qualified therapists. Even a brief visit or phone conversation may help you evaluate and resolve the problem.

If the employee dies, encourage co-workers to attend the funeral.

Being with others who are also grieving and listening to what family members and friends say about the person is an essential component of the grief process. Employees usually will benefit from participating in a ritual with others who cared about the person. To deprive them of this may cause problems later.

Sometimes employees want to conduct their own memorial service. Let the employees plan these services themselves. If they ask for your suggestions, you may want to encourage them to write down their memories of their co-worker, then read these aloud during the service. Employee memorial services that I have attended were held in auditoriums, offices, rose gardens, parks, and employees' homes.

If an employee is having an especially difficult time coping with a loss, encourage him to seek counseling. The organizations previously listed can refer you to a specialist. If the loss is seriously affecting the company, ask a professional therapist who consults with corporations to hold a meeting at the workplace where the employees can talk about their feelings.

SUPPORTING ABSENT EMPLOYEES

Find out if the employee wants to work at the hospital or at home.

Don't make any assumptions or try to guess how patients or caregivers feel about working away from the office. Instead, you may want to say, "I realize some people just want to focus on getting well when they are dealing with this disease, but others want to keep working. I want you to do what is best for you. I can bring you a computer or any other equipment you may need. If you change your mind or don't feel up to it, just let me know, and I would be happy to reassign the project."

Employees, both as patients and as caregivers, have spent many weeks working in hospitals. Caregivers set up laptop computers or small workstations in the corner of patients' rooms. Patients often found that working during a hospital stay was a good way to occupy their time. Both the nursing staff and the employers supported these arrangements. One nurse told me about a couple who worked together at the hospital. "It made them feel worthwhile," she said. "They had something to talk about besides the cancer, and it contributed to their positive attitude."

If your employee voices an interest in continuing to work, be specific when assigning a project to her. Make your expectations clear about what you want completed and when. Tell her to give you plenty of notice if she can't complete the project. Discuss it without imposing unreasonable expectations on her. You want her to feel included but not burdened.

When you call an employee who is ill, away from the office, ask if this is a good time to talk.

If you're calling to discuss the project he is working on, set a time to talk in advance. This will enable him to prepare for the conversation.

Even if you are a co-worker just calling to say hello, be sure to ask if it's a good time to talk. Sometimes employees do not want to hear from co-workers when they are ill. It may remind them of what they can't do or of how much they have to do. Other employees who are ill welcome the contact from their co-workers. It makes them feel connected, remembered, and part of the team.

Diane Blum offers a good rule for calling people: "I always say, 'Is this a good time? Do you have a few minutes?' "

For more ways to talk to an employee coping with cancer refer to Chapters 3 and 4 and to Chapter 6 if she is a primary caregiver.

PROVIDING EDUCATIONAL OPPORTUNITIES

Offer seminars.

Having a speaker from a cancer agency come to talk on a variety of topics will allow employees to feel more comfortable discussing health-related issues with their employers. It educates workers about a service that they may need now or in the future. Supervisors who organize these presentations foster a more open environment.

The speaker from the cancer agency does not have to discuss cancer specifically. More often than not, when I did presentations for companies on other topics like stress management, employees either came forth during the discussion or afterward with specific questions about cancer.

Attending these presentations can be a positive first step for employees. For those who used our agency afterward, they not only discovered a place to work out their cancer-related problems but were better able to concentrate at work than before. Resolving their cancer issues enabled them to pay more attention to their jobs while they were at the office.

Social worker Carolyn Messner, director of education and training at Cancer Care, explains that only speakers with training should do these presentations. They should be aware of the issues facing the employees and be able to relate to the audience. They should also know how to interject humor into a very heavy issue. They have to understand how to leave employees feeling upbeat and not depressed.

As Messner acknowledges: "The supervisor or person who arranges the seminar is on the line, accountable to make sure the speaker can deliver."

Before bringing a speaker into your company, attend one of her presentations, get recommendations from colleagues in the business community, or use a speakers' bureau.

Have a telephone consultation.

If you're the employer, call someone who has counseled employees on work-related issues. Call the NCI Cancer Information Service (800-4-CANCER) and ask for a referral to an agency in your area whose social workers or psychologists will talk to you about an employee. The resources listed at the end of the book will also provide individualized support.

Have an annual health fair and include cancer agencies.

Health fairs give employees a sense that their employer understands their needs. There they can learn about resources and meet experts in cancer care. This contact will allow them to feel more comfortable about calling an agency when they need support. They can also pick up educational brochures and mail them to friends and relatives.

A few weeks after I attended a health fair for Mobil, I received a call from Geoffrey, who lives in Louisiana. "I just wanted to thank you for this wonderful brochure, *I Have Cancer, This Is What You Can Do*. My brother obtained copies at the Mobil health fair and sent it out to my family. I have the disease, but I didn't know how to ask for help, and they didn't know how to support me until they read your brochure. Thanks to you, I have the assistance I need."

Guidelines for Co-Workers

Don't jump in and become a rescuer.

Too often, caring employees don't talk to patients or caregivers before unofficially taking it upon themselves to incorporate part of the co-worker's workload.

Soon, however, the employee may find that his own efficiency is affected. He will resent the co-worker he has tried to help if his own job suffers. If he had spoken to the person first, the problem could have been prevented.

Ask your co-worker how much he wants to discuss the situation.

If his illness is not interfering with his performance or affecting that of others, then it's up to him to decide how much he wants to share. Other than deciding on job responsibilities, certain patients and caregivers prefer never to talk about their personal lives at work. Others welcome the opportunity to share experiences. The only way to find out is to ask, "Is this something you want to discuss at work?" Or: "Is this a good time?" Or: "Do you mind if I ask how you're holding up, or would you rather I waited for you to tell me?" Or: "I'm sorry to hear about the cancer. Is it okay if I check in and see how you're doing, or would you prefer not to get too many questions?"

Ask your co-worker if she wants to assign a point person.

Ask her if she wants to assign one person to disseminate information to other workers. You could say to her, "Then you'll be free to initiate conversations about the disease when it's convenient. This will keep your day from being disrupted by questions from well-meaning co-workers."

Don't pull away.

More than fifty percent of patients with cancer will achieve a cure. Even if someone is going through a rough course of treatment, it may be temporary. Since cancer tends to be a long-term chronic illness, patients who have a poor prognosis can have hundreds of productive days.

If you pull away from a person who is coping with cancer, you are not only doing him a disservice, you are hurting yourself. His fighting spirit, whether he is a patient or a caregiver, may well raise office morale by inspiring others. He can teach co-workers how to put problems and priorities into perspective. He may have learned to look at situations from a more global view. Co-workers have a lot to learn from these employees; to avoid them is to miss out on valuable opportunities.

Many employers have shared stories about significant contributions that cancer patients and their loved ones made to their companies. But none stands out more than the one a volunteer made to my own business, Cancer Counseling, Inc.

While the volunteer, Bob Davis, was battling prostate cancer, he would call me with suggestions about how to improve CCI. One day he said, "You know what CCI needs? It needs a simple brochure to educate people about helping families with cancer. I'm going to write it."

I Have Cancer, This Is What You Can Do has been reprinted by *Coping* magazine, *Shell Oil Company News, The Candlelighter's Foundation,* and more than two hundred corporations, hospitals, civic groups, and cancer agencies. Almost a million copies, including reprints, have been distributed worldwide. Seven years later, it's still CCI's best educational pamphlet. Your company may have an employee like Bob, but you'll never know if you pull away from him.

Offer to find resources.

Offer to do research for your co-worker. Say, "I'd be happy to find out if there are any support groups or counselors who could help you through this tough time. Would you like me to look into it or get you educational brochures?"

Many employees are reluctant to call the human relations or personnel department or an in-house social worker because they don't want to discuss emotional issues with the company's staff. They have often called CCI after co-workers gave them our number. They always mentioned how grateful they were to the employees who had found this resource for them.

It's not your job to cheer the person up.

An executive with a computer company told me, "Every time I went by my assistant's desk, she made a comment about my expression. If I looked the least bit preoccupied, she made remarks like, 'You have to be positive.' 'Cheer up.' 'It's not that bad.'"

As a co-worker, you want to be compassionate to a colleague, but trying to cheer her up may not be the best way to show your concern. What patients and caregivers want, unless they say otherwise, is understanding. If you go out of your way to cheer them up, they may feel obligated to act happy *just to make you feel better.*

Keep conversations confidential.

Unless your co-worker specifically tells you that you can share what she's told you, assume you can't. If another employee or the supervisor asks you, "I noticed [the employee] talking to you. Can you tell me what is going on with her?" You should respond, "I'm sure she'll appreciate your concern, and I'll let her know you asked, but I'm not comfortable talking about what we discussed." Or: "I'm sorry, I can't reveal what she said, but you may want to let her know you're thinking about her by sending her a note or calling."

Don't say, "You're courageous."

When patients and loved ones are at work, they feel the extra burden of having to perform. Comments like this, however well intended, add to their already-tremendous stress.

Merry Templeton, from the American Cancer Society, recalled a woman who came to a support group. "The minute she walked in, she reached for her wig and threw it off. Then she said, 'I feel terrible, and it's so good to be here where I can say what I'm feeling. I am under so much pressure at work to live up to the praise my co-workers heap on me for handling the surgery so well. They make comments like 'You're so brave.' 'You look so great.' I know I don't look great—I can see it in the mirror. But I'm doing the best I can.

I'm wearing this wig to spare their feelings, to make it easier on them, because they can't deal with my bald head or the cancer. What I really want them to say is, 'I know you feel like hell. Please feel free to talk about it with me.' 'Tell me how you really feel.'"

Offer to help your co-worker on and off the job.

Employees who have projected a strong image at work may find it especially difficult to ask for assistance. Since you don't know how she feels about asking for help, you'll have to determine what kind of relationship you have with her before you ask if she wants your support.

Ask yourself, "What kind of relationship do we have?" The closer you are, the more you may want to become involved. On the other hand, if you've never paid attention to her before, it may appear hypocritical to hover over her suddenly, offering assistance.

If you're not sure how to approach her, write a note, indicating you are thinking about her and her family. If you want to help, list two or three things you are available to do.

Briefly stop by and *say* a few words. "I just wanted you to know I was thinking about you, and I'd like to help. I could do..."

Visit a patient at home or in the hospital, when it's appropriate.

Again, you'll have to decide whether your relationship warrants a visit, and you'll have to check and see if the person really wants visitors. If you don't want to go, don't. He will sense your reluctance if you do. Offer to visit only if you feel comfortable doing so.

Neal, a patient who endured nine months of chemotherapy and three weeks in the hospital, told me this story: "The most moving experience during that whole episode was a visit from Andy, a co-worker I barely knew.

"Andy had cancer, but he hadn't revealed it to anyone at work. He told me he felt he had something of value to share with me. He'd hoped he could serve as an example of a fellow traveler navigating a similar path.

"When Andy came to see me, he offered to answer any questions I had. I gladly accepted. But even if he didn't offer to talk about himself, his compassion and courage alone would have touched me."

Before you go, call the patient and ask him if he would like visitors. Say, "I'd like to come see you, but if you're not up to it, please tell me. Being in the hospital must be pretty difficult. We could arrange something afterward if that's more convenient." Most people will appreciate your offer, but some just don't want visitors from the office.

Maggie was upset because her husband wouldn't let anyone visit from his company. "They called and offered to come over, but Jake didn't want to see any of them, even those he was close to. He couldn't stand the idea of colleagues looking at him while he was sick. I didn't understand it, but I had to respect it. I just felt bad for his co-workers. I hope they understood it had nothing to do with them."

Send more than a group card.

Besides sending one group card, employees can each buy cards and write notes in them. Group cards are always great, but you should also send a personalized note or a simple card with a few lines in it if you're close to the person. One co-worker can put the cards in an envelope and hand-deliver them.

If the office is sending a gift, it's appropriate to attach a group card. Carolyn Messner recalls "an employee who got an enormous card from the staff. He was really touched by it."

One woman who had been hospitalized repeatedly for two years lamented, "All I ever got were group cards. I worked with six or seven of those employees for more than twenty years; had sent them many notes; bought them presents for special occasions; and had attended their weddings and other family events. If those employees, the ones I thought I was close to, even scribbled a few lines on toilet paper, it would have meant more than their signatures on group cards."

Send flowers and fun gifts.

Read Chapter 5 for ideas on gifts to send to your co-worker. Unless you are friends outside the workplace, give a simple gift, like a coffee cup, writing paper, a gift certificate, an upbeat novel, a cartoon you cut out, or a small framed picture.

When the person returns to work, don't overload her.

Carolyn Messner suggests you stop by and say hello or leave a note in the person's box, welcoming her back. "Then let the employee re-adjust without being bombarded by long conversations. Resume your normal way of interacting as soon as possible."

By following these guidelines, you and your company will achieve your goals while also gaining a powerful understanding of human behavior. You will learn skills that will be useful in any future challenges you face, both personally and professionally. Coping with illness in the workplace may seem like a huge burden at first. And it may be in many ways. Yet, if you address it openly and in a straightforward manner, it can become an opportunity to strengthen the employees' allegiance toward the company and each other.

Chapter 8

Giving Without Giving Out

Shannon will never forget that day—June 5 will be forever etched into her memory: "Tony seemed somewhat preoccupied, but rather calm considering where we were headed. He stared out across the highway as we navigated our way to his doctor's for the second visit. After a battery of tests at the medical center, Dr. Travis told us to come in. He had the test results.

"Tony appeared as though he could manage this force that was about to enter our lives. I, on the other hand, was in shock. No one had spoken the words yet, but I knew, as Tony probably did, that we were about to hear them.

"Once we arrived and were settled into the too-well-decorated lavender waiting room, I began to wonder, What's wrong with every-one else here? Are they worse off or better off than we're going to be?

"Eventually we found ourselves sitting in these high-back, dark blue Queen Anne chairs, facing an enormous glass-top desk, laid out with stacks of neatly ordered files. I remember thinking, Our lives are hidden somewhere among them.

"Then this tall, very handsome and distinguished man whisked into the room. I had grabbed the chair, clinging to it for strength. His presence terrified me; I knew his words alone could destroy our lives. The words he spoke only minutes later did just that."

A few months later Shannon described the changes in her life: "Just as I adjust to some aspects of this disease, others knock me over. I've read the pamphlets, the books, the articles. Tony has chosen a treatment. I feel as though I've entered this community. There's a camaraderie in the long winding hospital corridors we travel every day. We know some of the families by name, we know their stories, their pain. And the ones we've never met, we know them too.

"But I'm exhausted, and Tony's completely wrapped up in himself, lost in a place where I cannot reach him. He does not notice me. It's as though I've disappeared, replaced by this disease. And his calm demeanor has left us too. He doesn't appreciate my constant care. If I even mention my needs, he yells, 'But I'm the one with cancer.'"

A few months later a different Shannon talked about the illness: "We've joined a couples' group, and the therapist and members have helped us handle some of our problems. I'm learning how to juggle it all, but I'm not sure that's a good thing.

"Tony's angry phase has settled permanently into our home. My kids are always complaining, sometimes at him but more often than not at me. Some days all I want to do is walk out the door and never come back. I know it seems selfish, but it is so hard to live this way."

A year later, Shannon had incorporated most of the suggestions in the next two chapters of this book. "If I had my choice, I'd have booted this disease out of our lives. But I didn't have that choice. What I did have was the power to control the things I could and to let go of those I couldn't. Life will never hand us back our innocence or safety nets. But our relationships are better than I ever imagined they could be. To get here took practice and scrapes and nicks and cuts and arguments and tears.

"I respect my needs as well as his. I take care of myself. I treasure who and what I am. Tony shares his feelings instead of withdrawing or taking them out on me.

"We still have a long way to go. I doubt we will ever actually arrive in some safe haven, but the journey is full of lessons. I now embrace those I've learned as well as those that lie ahead.

"Tony still battles the ravages of this disease, and there are times when I feel so helpless against the force that he faces. But we're in this together now, and together we can tackle whatever God throws our way."

The mixed emotions, the roller-coaster ride, that Shannon experienced are common among people facing a long-term illness. This chapter addresses ways anyone can manage the roller coaster. As Lucy Kim, the wife of a patient, whom we met in Chapter 5, said, "In 1989 I learned these methods, and I still use them today. The good thing about learning many different techniques is that you have a reserve to turn to in a crisis. When you are in the middle of an emergency or having a really hard time, you cannot think of how to overcome it. But if you learn ways to deal with it before it happens, then you can easily apply them. If one doesn't work, you can try another. You have a whole reserve of ammunition to throw at the problem. Before I had these as a safety net, it took longer and was more difficult to get through the tough days."

Risks to Your Health

Studies dating back to the 1970s looked for a correlation between stress caused by life crises and subsequent illness. Sixty percent of those with high stress levels were physically ill within eighteen months. But the other 40 percent, who had equally high stress levels, did not get sick. Why?

Some researchers speculate that the difference is due to biological factors—genes. In addition, the 40 percent may have handled the challenges in their lives in ways that promoted good health. A catastrophic illness is fraught with challenges, obstacles, and disappointments. You need to navigate through these while staying in the best physical and emotional shape you can. Otherwise you won't be good to yourself, the patient, or anyone else.

In order to avoid becoming one of the 60 percent, you have to treat yourself like an athlete headed into a marathon. By preparing yourself, building your inner strengths, and utilizing outside support, you will have a better chance of remaining healthy.

"But I Don't Have Time."

One wife sums up the feelings of many: "But I'm fine. It's the patient who is sick. I'm too busy. I'll take care of myself when this *passes*."

Unfortunately, a catastrophic disease rarely *passes*. In the best scenario the patient will achieve remission, only to be faced with years of checkups and fears of recurrence. Your marathon has only just begun—you need to start paying attention to your needs now, even if it seems as if you don't have the time.

But how do you take care of yourself? I touched briefly on a few ways in Chapter 2, including writing about your feelings, reaching out to others, celebrating smaller victories, laughing, and taking time to regroup.

Another way to increase your chances of remaining healthy is to resolve the issues that interfere with living life to its fullest.

Live the Just-in-Case Lifestyle

The realities of catastrophic illness are hard to face, especially when the patient is terminal. There's an enormous impetus toward denial, toward not facing the worst of outcomes. Denial is understandable, but there are some issues that you and your loved one must resolve nonetheless. If you don't, they'll permeate other areas of your life and affect your ability to function.

Dr. Norman Decker, of Baylor College of Medicine, advances the "just-in-case approach." He sees it as "a way to hold two mutually contradictory ideas in your mind as reality, either simultaneously or alternately. For example, the doctors might find a cure for the cancer (one idea), but 'just in case' it doesn't work (the second idea), you put your affairs in order. You take care of living wills, powers of attorney, and financial business, and you talk to your children."

If you use this approach, you can maintain realistic dreams and hopes for the future while ensuring that if they are not fulfilled, you are prepared. Every member of one of my couples groups revised their wills. As the husband of one patient reflected: "My wife wanted us to update our legal documents. I thought she was silly, but in the back of my mind, I was worrying about our affairs being in order. Once we handled these issues, we were able to concentrate on living. We don't waste energy thinking about providing for our kids, because we've taken care of it already. We are prepared *just in case* something happens."

When illness strikes, you have no idea what tomorrow will hold. You never did anyway, but the disease shatters the illusion that tomorrow will always arrive. A serious illness puts a lid not only on the patient's life but also over your dreams and visions for the future. To take off the lid, you must develop a new vision of where you want to go.

Doria, a hospital research assistant, had wanted to attend medical school. She hadn't even applied when her husband discovered he had cancer. Together they decided that she would try to fulfill her vision anyway, as best she could.

She had to take detours, and alter her short-term plans, when her husband was hospitalized for long periods of time, but she never gave up her dream. Today Doria is a much-loved, very respected doctor in a midwestern hospital.

Abigail was making huge strides in her career, when her husband, Henry, was diagnosed with a rare form of cancer. At thirty-four she suddenly understood that the plan she had made to have a baby would never be realized if they didn't try before Henry started his chemotherapy. But Henry suggested that they freeze his sperm, then wait and see how the treatment progressed before trying to become parents.

At first, Abigail was furious that Henry wasn't willing to try to have a child immediately. "After all, he already has three boys from his previous marriage, but I have no children of my own," Abigail said. "I didn't think it was too much to ask, given that I was willing and financially able to support a child as well as Henry."

Six months into the treatment, Henry changed his mind. He was handling the treatment well, and regardless of the outcome, he decided he ought to let Abigail try to fulfill her vision of motherhood.

Eight years later, Henry stopped by my office. Seven-year-old Charlie was tugging at his sleeve. "I think it's this little man whose helped me beat the odds," Henry said. "I can't imagine life without him."

Spring break had come early. The damp cold—worse sometimes than the fifteen below I've felt in Wyoming—had all but disappeared, replaced by perfect days, which in Houston, are few and far between. We were sitting around at the beginning of one of my couples' groups, talking about the welcomed breezes, budding azaleas, and blooming trees and how we were going to celebrate the spring holidays.

Hunter, who was always thinking ahead, said, "Since I just found out I have cancer, we didn't have much time to plan for spring. So how about if we talk about what we're going to do next summer?" Eliza, who had been told she had less than three months to live, looked over at Hunter, straightened her back, and proudly announced, "I'm going to Europe with my son, Ryan. We've already started planning the trip.

"I know what you're thinking," she added, "I won't make it. But that's okay too. We have enjoyed reading brochures, talking to others, and studying European history."

Shane, her husband, smiled. "It makes me feel good when I pass the den, and they are huddled over scattered brochures and books and magazine clippings. I know now that even if this monster interferes with their plans, they have spent more precious time together than ever before. That's what is really important."

Visions don't always materialize. But they do give you a goal to strive for, something positive to look forward to. Your vision may be as simple as reaching a certain level at a sport, spending summers with your family, or traveling across an ocean. Whatever it is, it can become your foundation, the source of strength to carry you through the most difficult days. "Do everything you can to go on living. Do whatever it takes to fulfill your concept of happiness," advises Dr. Lamar McGinnis, a past president of the American Cancer Society.

Start making your vision real by devising long-term plans and short-term goals. Compile a list of the benefits and rewards that you'll achieve by fulfilling your dream. After evaluating the list, you may discover very quickly that it's not your dream after all, or you may become even more committed to fulfilling your vision.

The vision should accommodate who you are and not what other people think you should be. You should approach the plan with realistic optimism. Stay positive and hopeful, but be realistic about the patient's limitations as well as her interests.

Break up the long-term vision into achievable short-term goals. You should always strive to reach your ultimate dream, but enjoy the process of attaining it as well. When you work toward your dream in stages, planning will seem less overwhelming.

While planning each stage, include ways to take care of yourself as well as the patient that meet both of your needs physically, emotionally, socially, and spiritually. By enjoying the stages and rewarding yourself as you accomplish goals, you make each day more rewarding than if you wait only to enjoy your final dreams.

Whether you keep a daily to-do list or a calendar, keep track of whether you are achieving your short-term goals.

Create a list of ways you can reward yourself as you attain them. Think about what makes you feel good, what treats you can give yourself. It can range from a pat on the back to a few hours of fun. Have you ever achieved something you really felt good about? Did your parents or someone else say something about this accomplishment that added to your excitement? After you meet a goal, say those same words to yourself.

Your plans have to be flexible. Be willing to cancel events and projects at a moment's notice if an emergency arises with the patient's health or in any other area of your life. Initially, you may resent making last-minute changes. But making them teaches you skills that can help you overcome disappointments and adapt to change. Given the number of changes we all undergo throughout our lives, these skills are invaluable.

Don't Go It Alone

Seek out friends who can and will support you in taking care of yourself. Spend time with people who will help you discover the positive aspects of your life, who make you feel good about yourself, who bring humor into your life, and who will listen when you're down.

The people you spend time with should be those who accept you as you are. The difficulty is you may have expected certain friends to be supportive, only to discover they can't be. Be sure to have others who will stand by you.

Out of tragedy can come blessings. As one wife of a patient said, "Two positive aspects of the disease are the friends we've made and the friendships we've learned to appreciate and treasure. I'd never have believed this could come out of such a horrible experience."

Try to contact friends you've lost touch with. Some people may be afraid to call you. (Chapter 2 will give you insights into why.) They may not know how to support you. Call those once-close friends who are now absent. If they don't call back, then you will have to let go of these friends for now, and maybe forever. One of the greatest tragedies of this disease is the loss of friendships. The pain associated with these losses can last for years. But I can assure you that by doing some of the activities in this chapter, you will make new friends.

Whether or not your friends are there for you, find a trained volunteer, a support group, or a professional counselor to talk with. A well-run group is a safe, nonjudgmental place to discuss your concerns. You don't have to talk about yourself—you can just listen to how others cope. Robert, the neurologist whose wife has cancer, describes his couples' group, "It allows me to listen to the ways others deal with their marriages, their children, and the cancer. When I hear another spouse talk about a marital problem, I'm more willing to listen than if my wife brought up the same issue. I can hear the problem discussed without feeling like the comments are directed at me."

His wife, Sue, adds, "I want to tell him how I'm feeling, but there are times when I'm not very good at articulating my thoughts. Then someone in the group explains the same issue in a way Robert can understand. I also get ideas about how to talk about the cancer with him, ways I would never have thought of on my own."

One group member thanked Robert for his participation. "When you talk, it clarifies my issues. When you listen to me and ask questions, it also helps me see my problems from a different point of view."

Here are some other benefits people have found in counseling, either in individual sessions or in a support group:

> "Two of the closest friends I have today are men I met eight years ago in my support group."
> "Individual and family counseling was the guide through the valley of death. It helped us take our muddled thoughts and turn them into concrete deeds, convert our anxieties into positive action, focus on our real problems, and then take steps to solve them."
> "I needed someone to listen. You don't always have people who want to listen to you after fighting this disease for so many years."
> "I learned new ways of dealing with uncertainties, and I knew the group was a safe harbor, regardless of the medical prognosis."
> "In just two meetings I took comfort from the fact that others understood what I was feeling at two A.M."

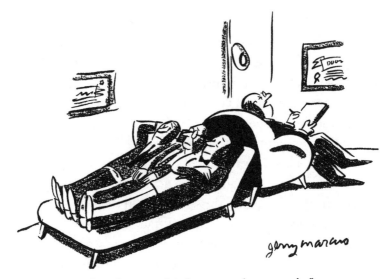

"First, let me explain how group therapy works."

Reprinted with permission from The Saturday Evening Post Society/a division of the BFL & MS, Inc. © 1984.

The following is a list of organizations that will give you referrals to volunteer or professional counselors. When you call one of the professional resources, say, "I'm looking for a social worker, psychologist, or psychiatrist who has at least five years of experience working with families coping with cancer. Can you give me the names of three people to whom you have referred before? Can you tell me a little bit about each one?" Additional organizations can be found in the Resources section of this book.

- A local medical school's psychiatric clinic or department of psychiatry
- A clinical psychology or social work department at a local university
- The American Psychiatric Association, (202) 682-6000
- The American Psychological Association, (202) 336-5700. The APA will refer you to your state psychological association, which will provide you with referrals to members in your area.

- The National Association of Social Workers, (202) 408-8600
- The National Family Caregivers Association, (800) 896-3650. If you join, you can receive their quarterly newsletter *Take Care!* and become a member of their network, which links caregivers to others in similar situations.
- The social work department at the hospital you used for treatment
- Your local United Way

When caring for your loved one becomes too overwhelming, you must get help yourself. Seek professional support, no matter what, if you have these warning signs:

You feel overwhelmed.

You can't sleep.

You have changed your eating habits, leading to a radical change in weight. Dr. Norman Decker recommends, "If, without your conscious intent, you gain or lose more than ten pounds, something is seriously wrong."

You cannot concentrate at work.

You have a sense of despair or suicidal feelings.

You are experiencing anxiety attacks.

You haven't been to the doctor in over a year.

You've withdrawn from friends and family.

You're drinking more or abusing drugs.

You're too busy to talk to friends whom you cared about before.

You feel like an accident waiting to happen, or you're having numerous accidents.

You know about ways to take care of yourself but never have time to implement them.

You feel tired all the time.

You feel as if there is not one positive thing in your life that you can count on.

Understand and Compromise: Getting Along with Others

A few weeks after he finished radiation, Matthew withdrew emotionally from his wife, Jessica. Jessica explained it this way: "Matthew isn't a talker, at least when it comes to problems he can't fix right away. He's a pilot by training. Everything is mechanical, even emotional problems."

Matthew explained his withdrawal, "I need time to figure out my problems in my head before I talk about them with others."

Jessica didn't understand that for Matthew, dealing with the cancer by himself was helpful. "I just think he doesn't want to work on the emotional issues we're facing," she said. "He doesn't pay attention when I talk to him. It's like he immediately switches off if he senses I'm going to mention anything to do with the emotional aspects of the disease."

"I do switch off," Matthew replied to her, "because I can't think when you get irrational. I am trying to figure it out, but I need my solitude to do that."

Jessica had yet to understand that Matthew's way of dealing with problems was different from hers. Matthew, for his part, had to find a way to share his feelings with her.

They came to my group to work out their problems. We asked Matthew if he would be willing to set up an hour or two to talk about Jessica's concerns with her, after he had had a reasonable amount of time to sort things out on his own. He agreed to meet with her the night before their next session.

It wasn't easy for Jessica to be quiet and patient and respect his wishes. It made her feel helpless and useless. During the group session the next day, Matthew told the group, "Jessica and I shared our feelings. It went very well because we waited until I was comfortable."

If your coping style is different from that of your loved one, you still need to have your needs met. Call a friend or a counselor, or attend a group, if your loved one withdraws from you. Until he is ready to talk, seek out friends who listen well and acknowledge your feelings.

It is hard not to take it personally when someone doesn't treat you as you would wish, even if that person is sick. It is especially hard when you are in close contact with the person. Sometimes every word, every look, seems like a direct attack. He may be so wrapped up in his own world that he is not appreciative of yours. He may not even realize that his words are having a negative impact on you.

Sometimes you just have to ask the patient to provide what you need. Jessica discovered that when she used the following statements, Matthew paid more attention to her needs:

> "Sometimes I need you to tell me how I'm doing. I need feedback. I need to know if you like how I'm fixing your meals or making up your room."
> "I sometimes have feelings that I'm not doing enough, that I'm not doing it the right way, or that I'm doing all this work and you don't even notice."
> "It would make me feel better if you said . . ."

Master the Dynamics of Anger: Yours and Your Loved One's

Anger can drive even the closest people apart. When illness strikes, there are many things that people get angry about. Here are a few things that patients and loved ones have said they were mad at. They may help you to understand your own anger, as well as any anger that is directed toward you:

> "The cancer itself, the new responsibilities, people, the losses, and the limited choices."
> "Each other's way of handling the disease."
> "The policies of the insurance company, the employer, or the government."
> "Life in general."
> "My wife's behavior triggers feelings from the past, and I get angry."

Take a pencil right now and write down five things you are mad at. Repeat this exercise whenever you notice that you're raising your voice, clenching your fists, or feeling aggravated.

Here are some other techniques for dealing with anger:

Use visualization.

Whenever either of you is attacking the other, try to stand back. Visualize the fight as a movie. Picture a tiny director in your head as he asks you: "Where are we going with this?" "What is this going to accomplish?" "Is this really worth fighting over?"

Every time you argue, take two minutes. Think about your director. Have him stop you. This may be difficult at first. Hopefully with practice it can become a habit, a tool that enables you to be more objective and less emotional.

Talk to yourself, and translate the meaning.

Dr. Decker suggests you hold a running dialogue with yourself. "Continually tell yourself that hostile comments have nothing to do with you. Say: 'This is not really about me. This is about my wife's disease, or her feelings about the disease.'

"You have to translate the person's comments. It's not always easy. When someone kicks you in the shins, it still hurts, regardless of why she kicked you."

Be empathetic, not defensive.

You're better off reacting to anger in an empathetic way. If you respond by being angry and defensive, the fight will most likely escalate.

Lower and relax the tone of your voice.

The louder her voice gets, the quieter and calmer you need to become. Although it sometimes feels great to yell back, you usually pay for it later.

Lowering your voice, staying calm, and being understanding will defuse a great deal of the hostility. Also, relax your shoulders, put your hands in a comfortable position, and take three deep breaths. It's harder for people to yell at someone who appears peaceful and understanding.

Be compassionate, and consider the contributing factors.

Remember how Eliza, from Chapter 4, described what she was facing? "I'm dealing with losing everyone and everything I know," she said. Think about how you would feel if this were happening to you. Even a patient with a curable disease experiences so many physical, spiritual, and emotional assaults that she may lash out in anger.

Certain medications can also spark reactions that patients aren't completely in control of. When one of my patients was on morphine and recovering from surgery, he was nasty to his adult children. Today he doesn't even remember their visit.

Don't blame.

When either you or your loved one is angry, avoid blaming each other. Blaming is saying that you're right and he's wrong. Appearing "right" is a way of dominating someone else. Little good can come out of such a rigid stance.

Don't hit below the belt.

It may feel good at the time, but if you care about the person, you'll feel awful later. Below-the-belt comments can stay with your loved one for months, even years. Often these comments are based on information that you've probably learned about in intimate situations. If you use this information to hurt, you are setting up an unending pattern of distrust.

Say you are sorry.

When you've started an argument or escalated one, apologize.

Watch out for attack statements.

"You are..." "If only you would..." "If you don't do it, then I'll..." Avoid making these kinds of coercive and threatening remarks.

Focus on what you or the person can change.

Don't focus on things or people you can't change. Avoid making statements like "If this hadn't happened to begin with..." and "If you didn't..." and "If only..." It has happened, and things are the way they are. Now how are you going to deal with the situation?

Do not allow yourself to be abused.

Leave the room if you or your loved one can't control the anger. You're not running away—you're conserving energy to tackle the issue when the intensity of the situation is defused. Before you leave, say:

> "I need to stop this conversation. I don't want us to
> hurt each other. Let's continue this when we're not so
> upset."
> "It's hard for me to listen now. Maybe we can talk
> about this later when I've calmed down, because I'm
> getting really upset."
> "I care about you. I love you. I don't want to fight with
> you. Can we talk about this later, when we have a
> better perspective? I don't want to say things I don't
> mean."

Anger is associated with major life changes, but abuse and violence are not acceptable ways to express it.

Use brief caring statements to defuse an argument.

"It makes me angry or afraid when you talk
that way."

"I want to work this out with you. If you could
be specific about what you want or what's wrong,
then I could understand your point of view
better."

"I love you. Can we find a way to discuss this
that makes us both feel good? We already feel bad
enough about the cancer. That's my real enemy,
not you."

Use anger to fuel your energy in a positive direction.

You can use anger as fuel to gain control over your situation in positive ways. Jenna was mad at her husband's family. "When they came
to see him, they stomped right over me, expecting me to cater to
them. Could I bring them something to eat or get the *TV Guide* or
move furniture around to make *them* comfortable? They wouldn't
dream of asking me if they could help him. They thought their visits
were help enough. As if I should be *grateful* that they graced us with
their presence! And they berated me for how I took care of him.
Nothing I did was ever right."

Finally Jenna exploded. Fortunately, it was during one of our sessions and not one of their visits. Taking the advice of the other group
members, Jenna read some books on being assertive. She practiced
the tips they suggested and began to incorporate them into her
behavior.

Eventually she became assertive with her husband's parents. They
respected her attitude. "Can you believe they even asked me how they
could help?" Jenna used her newly acquired skills with doctors, insurance representatives, and anyone else who would have previously
upset her.

As Rabbi Roy Walter of Temple Emanu El, in Houston, says, "You
have choices about anger. You can swallow it, leave it as it is, or you can

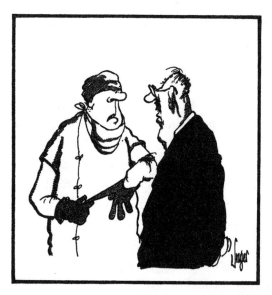

**"Your wife is still under the anesthetic
and, from what I've heard,
this would be a good time to see her."**

Copyright © Jim Unger/dist. by Laughingstock. Herman® comics by Jim Unger were reprinted with
the permission of Laughingstock Licensing, Inc.

deal with it. Even when you're angry at God, acknowledge it. When
you have a relationship, you can be angry and still love someone." As
Dr. Decker and I used to advise our clients, "God has big shoulders.
He can handle your anger."

Once you release your anger, several things may happen. You
may discover you weren't angry at all. You may be able to forgive the
person. You may learn to replace the anger with acceptance or you
may decide that the anger doesn't serve a purpose and won't change
anything.

Handling Unwanted Advice

When someone gives you unsolicited advice, acknowledge their
desire to help and use what you can. Say:

"I'm grateful for your support. Let me think about
   that."
"I hear what you're saying, but I'm not sure if it will
   work for me. I'll consider it."
"I appreciate your ideas, but in this case I need to do
   it this way. I hope you understand."
"You know, that is interesting. I never thought about
   it that way. I'll keep it in mind."
"I'm not sure whose way will help the patient more, so
   let's compromise so we can provide the best support."
"Let's discuss this with the patient. He can tell us the
   best way we can help him, because I'm not sure what
   he needs."

Dr. Lamar McGinnis encourages you to "discount any information that is based on hearsay or untruths." Relatives may try to help resolve a conflict, but without knowing the whole story, they may be basing their advice on experiences very different from yours.

People who offer unsolicited advice often are those who feel out of control, helpless, or anxious. The only way they can regain control is to offer opinions. By acknowledging their suggestion, then cutting the conversation short or changing the subject, you enable them to maintain their dignity.

Practice Time Management

An important part of taking care of yourself and your family is managing your time efficiently. The next section gives you ideas about ways other people coping with cancer have organized their lives.

Whether you work at home or at an office, keep a to-do list in a daily Day-Timer or in a pocket-size electronic organizer. Start each day by writing down projects you have to complete, calls you have to make, and appointments you need to keep that day. Throughout the morning and afternoon, check off tasks as you complete them, whenever possible.

Before you go home, check off any other projects, calls, or tasks you completed in the afternoon. Move items you couldn't finish to the beginning of the next day's list or to another day. You may decide the item can wait for a few weeks, or you may want to delete it altogether. Marking off items and keeping your tasks organized will give you a sense of accomplishment and order.

Everyone has strengths and weaknesses. Put a star on your to-do list by the items that involve your weaknesses and delegate them if you can. Think of people who could take on these chores—friends, family members, or volunteers. Write their names by the star. Then call them and ask for their help.

Let's say you hate to cook. Whenever you have to prepare dinner, you storm around the kitchen banging pans and slamming drawers. You have been wonderful to the patient for days, helped her in more ways than most husbands ever would. But now you're upset, and she can hear you storming around the kitchen. Unfortunately, anything else you do for her will be overshadowed by your anger.

If you hate to do something, find someone else to do it. If family or friends won't help, then call United Way and ask which of their agencies has volunteers. If no one can help, then hire a college or high school student for a nominal fee to do whatever you can delegate. Don't be put off if the student doesn't do the job as well as you would have. The goal is not to have everything completed perfectly, but to allow you to focus on the chores you have to do, the ones you enjoy, and the ones you do best.

If you are taking care of a sibling or parent, then hold a family meeting. Have ready a list of all the jobs required to take care of the patient. Say, "This is what has to be done. This is what I can do. Let's find a way to split the rest of the chores."

If they don't live nearby, hold the meeting by telephone conference. An operator can organize this for you. At the very least the family may be willing to send money to pay for someone else to do the services the patient needs. Family members can also help you find resources by calling private or government agencies. They can gather information and send you brochures and forms.

Too often adult children who become caregivers take on more than they can handle, trying to maintain their own lives as well as their parents. An ill parent may move in and become the focus of an adult child's life, at the expense of the spouse and children. If this sounds like you, you need to set boundaries and delegate tasks. Suppose your father lived in another state or refused to move in with you. In that case you would be forced to find some way to get him resources. You'd have to. Unfortunately, when someone lives close by, doing everything yourself becomes a habit or is simply easier. Next time you offer to help, imagine the person lives far away. Stop and ask yourself whom you would call for help. That same resource may be available to you right now, in your own city.

Shanna's mother lives in Montana and loves it. When she was ill, she didn't want to leave her friends. So her daughter took a week off, went up to Montana, and arranged for all the services her mother needed. While Shanna was there, she investigated other services that her mother might need in the future, like the senior center, Meals on Wheels, and a rehabilitation center. She gathered business cards from staff members and volunteers and made their acquaintance in case she had to call them in the future. It has been six years since Shanna first went to Montana. Her mother has used not only the original services her daughter arranged but many of the other services, such as the senior center.

Dr. Ernest Katz, director, Behavioral Sciences Section, Children's Center for Hematology-Oncology, Children's Hospital Los Angeles, summarizes his concerns about family members as primary caregivers and the problems they face if they don't learn to delegate. "It is essential for caregivers to have a balanced life," he says. "I'm very cautious about people who are overly devoted to their work [for patients]. They can't really be effective. Many times people like that lose their boundaries. They may seem extremely compassionate, but the patients they are trying to help may perceive them as a burden. As caregivers, we need to recognize we are there to help people throughout pain and tragedy. We can't personalize the entire experience. We also have to have our own healthy relationships."

If you completely devote yourself to the patient, you may lose focus on your own life. Before you fall into the Supercaregiver trap, get a piece of paper and pencil and answer these questions:

- Am I trying to do this all myself because I was taught I have to?
- What benefits—emotional or social—do I derive from worrying about nothing but the patient? What am I getting out of doing it all myself?
- Are there parts of my own life I am ignoring or neglecting? Which ones? Why?
- Would I be more helpful and more effective if I found others to help me?
- Am I afraid to delegate? What is the worst that could happen if I asked others to help me?
- If I could find others to help, what would I do with the free time I would then have?

Delegating is essential to your well-being, and to that of your loved one. If your loved one senses that you are overburdened, she may feel guilty, angry, or sad, or she may stop telling you what her needs are so as not to burden you further. What you want is an open, caring relationship. To achieve this, you may have to reevaluate how you are caring for her. Have a discussion with her about how she perceives you as a caregiver.

Another delegating technique is to keep a shopping list in a place where everyone who either works in your house or lives there can add items to it. Ask family members and household help to write items on the list throughout the week. This turns over to them the responsibility for keeping track of their own needs, and it prevents you from having to run out to the store every other day, which wastes time and depletes energy.

Another way to take care of yourself is to research the available services that the patient may need in the future. Ask the patient's doctor or nurse what services may become necessary. A hospital social worker can often guide you through this maze of services and help you to complete the forms.

Once the doctor has decided on a treatment for your loved one, call the insurance company or the government (for Medicaid and Medicare) to inquire about coverage and completing the forms. Explain what services you think you will be needing, such as equipment or home health services. Ask if the agency can send forms now, so you don't have to fill them out during a crisis. Sometimes one coverage expires, and it takes weeks to apply for the next type of coverage. And the government may require copies of bank statements and other legal documents that take time to acquire.

Keeping an organized file cabinet will save you hours of looking for documents. Your file cabinet can be as simple as a box large enough to hold legal-size folders. The first section should be for your blank paper:

- *Letterhead stationery and envelopes.* Have your name, address, and phone and fax numbers printed on the letterhead. Copying centers and office supply stores will print stationery in quantities of up to five hundred for a minimal charge. This will save you hours of addressing correspondence.
- *Thank-you supplies.* If you write numerous thank-you notes, set up a file folder containing your personalized stationery.

Next, make categories for the major areas you deal with routinely, such as doctors, bills, and receipts. Using color-coded labels, set up a section for each category in alphabetical order, designating a color for each section. Within each section file the folders in alphabetical order. For example:

- **Doctor bills**—blue. Using blue labels, put folders with the doctors' last names into alphabetical order.

- **H**ospitals, nursing care, and clinics—yellow.
- **L**egal documents and copies—brown. The originals should be in a safe-deposit box.
- **R**eceipts—orange. Include receipts for pharmaceuticals, parking, and any other expense that your loved one may be able to deduct on her taxes.
- **S**ocial service agencies—red.
- **T**hird-party payers—blue. Include insurance companies, Medicaid, and Medicare. Make copies of documents you send to the insurance company or government, in case they get lost.
- **W**ish list. This is a list of tasks you need completed. Refer to it whenever someone calls and volunteers to help. Write his name by whatever project he agrees to do. Keep unmarked copies of this list. Give them to people who will coordinate help. For example, if one neighbor wants to organize help from your neighborhood, give her the list and let her schedule neighbors to cook, shop, and drive your kids to school.

Attach notes to bills, briefly describing any conversations you have had about problems with them. Each time you talk to someone about a bill, write his name and the date on it. Add one or two lines about what you agreed would happen as a result of your conversation. If a question arises later, you'll have a record of the commitments the person made to you. File the most recent bills in front, working backward.

Another time management technique is to schedule when *you* want to talk on the phone. Then turn on your answering machine the rest of the time. This arrangement will enable you to regroup and enjoy yourself, either alone or with your family. If you jump as soon as the phone rings, you are never going to have those much-needed, uninterrupted, rejuvenating moments.

Finally, don't waste time questioning your decisions. Once you've made a decision, let it go. Under these conditions it's too easy to be hard on yourself. Have confidence that given what you know today, you have made the best choice. If circumstances change, you can alter your course of action. Until you do, have confidence in your decision-making abilities.

Build In Ways to Be Good to Yourself

COMPARTMENTALIZE YOUR STRESSFUL THOUGHTS

Set aside time each day or at the very least once a week to reflect on the disease, its problems, its challenges, and its meaning to you. You can do this by writing about it, by talking to friends, and/or by meditating. Structuring this time will keep you from obsessing about the disease. Obsessive thinking rarely solves any problems and it drains you.

Robert, the neurologist from Chapter 1, refers to himself as "a habitual obsessor." He couldn't sleep at night because he would toss and turn, going over and over his wife's cancer in his head: "How can I get more information? Whom can I call? Why did the doctor say that? Why is my wife acting this way? What is she not telling me?" During the daytime he was distracted by the cancer. If he was out with others, he'd steer the conversation to the disease, and he wouldn't listen when friends discussed other subjects. His mind was always wandering, always returning to his wife's illness.

Finally he realized he had to stop obsessing, since he wasn't functioning. He learned how to compartmentalize his cancer thoughts, setting aside time each week to focus on the disease, to give it his full, undivided attention. "Every time I obsessed about the disease," he says, "I stopped and told myself to *save those thoughts* for the time I had scheduled for reflection—Tuesday afternoons. I visualized putting those thoughts in a box, knowing I could open it later. It's not always possible to set aside your emotions, but this technique reduced the amount of time I spent worrying. When Tuesday afternoons came, I gave my full attention to the cancer and my thoughts and feelings about it. Sometimes I called a friend and talked, releasing the emotions that way. Sometimes I wrote in my journal, and sometimes I just took a long walk and reflected on our situation."

Initially many people are afraid to join a support group. They think they will become even more obsessed with their problems than they already are. As one woman said, "Why should I go somewhere to talk about my problems for ninety minutes every week? That seems awfully negative." Yet she was spending at least seventy percent of every day thinking about her problems. After a few months in a support group, she went "from focusing on the cancer seventy percent of the day," she said, "to probably twenty percent. When I obsessed over it, I didn't resolve anything, and I wasted precious time. Now I talk about my issues once a week in a constructive manner during group. I'm able to look at the cancer and the changes in my life and evaluate them in a way that helps me feel more in control of my life."

Compartmentalizing your thoughts takes practice. If you find your mind wandering to the disease more than fifty percent of the day, the following exercise may help you: For three weeks set aside forty to sixty minutes at a time to think or talk about the illness. During this time attend a support group, call a friend, or go somewhere by yourself. At the end of three weeks, you should be spending more time focusing on living and less on worrying about the disease.

SCHEDULE ENJOYMENT

During one of the times you have set aside, evaluate how you can build enjoyment into your life. Ask yourself these questions:

- What do I like to do?
- If I had an extra two hours this week, how would I spend them?
- How did I formerly spend free time?
- Which activities could I still do if I had two hours free?
- Do I need to spend more time with others, or do I need time alone?
- Would I derive more joy from visiting people or from talking to them by phone?

Write down ten things you would do if someone said, "You have two hours to yourself today." Pick one of them, and do it once a week.

Schedule it by blocking in time for it on your calendar, just as you would any other appointment.

USE RELAXATION TECHNIQUES

Another way to improve your well-being is to learn methods for relaxation and make them part of your daily routine. Every day for thirty minutes, practice relaxation, or take a "brain break." Dr. Norman Decker recommends: "Do something that significantly reduces your anxiety level once a day. It ought to become a habit, like brushing your teeth. Listening to a progressive relaxation tape for thirty minutes will have a carryover effect for the rest of the day. Once you get good at relaxing, you can plug in the tape when you are anxious and relax easily."

Other ways to learn relaxation include:

- Call your local Transcendental Meditation organization and learn those techniques.
- Buy *The Relaxation Response* by Herbert Benson and study his methods of relaxation.
- Contact the Association for Applied Physiology and Feedback and the Biofeedback Certification Institute of America for a referral to someone who can train you in biofeedback techniques. Both organizations can be reached at (303) 422-8436 or www.aapb.org.
- Pay a therapist to teach you biofeedback.
- Call the American Council of Hypnotist Examiners, (800) 494-9766 or www.hypnosisforhealth.com. ACHE provides referrals to qualified practitioners and offers a catalog of relaxation tapes.
- Make your own relaxation tape by recording exercises by someone recommended by ACHE or a cancer agency. Therapists from some non-profit agencies will make you a tape at no charge. An ACHE-referred trained hypnotist will also help you make a personalized tape. You bring the recorder and tape the

relaxation exercise. Sometimes it may take two visits, but you will have the tape for years.

- Buy the book *Rituals of Healing: Using Imagery for Health and Wellness,* by Jeanne Achterberg, Barbara Dossey, and Leslie Kolkmeir. This book contains numerous easy-to-follow relaxation exercises.
- Use music to relax you. A music therapist may be available through your local hospital. Therapists who work with patients often have training to work with caregivers as well.
- Combat tension by taking three breaths. Nurse Mary Hughes suggests: "If you're clutching your hand or gritting your teeth, or if your shoulders are tense, then something's going on. Combat this tension by taking three deep breaths, and then relax."
- Do the squeeze-release-tension exercise. Grip something close by—like a steering wheel or a chair—or press your hands together. Squeeze as hard as you can, then relax. Visualize all the tension going to the place you are gripping. As you let go, picture the tension drifting toward the sky like a balloon. Repeat as many times as you need to until you feel relaxed.
- Go to a place of worship. Sit quietly. Pray, or have a conversation with Whomever you pray to. You can also go to this sanctuary in your mind. Sit back and visualize yourself walking into this place. Picture the walls, the solitude, the quietness. Then with your eyes closed, do the same things you would do if you were in a place of worship.

READ

Reading is also a good way to regroup, relax, and escape. A good book is like a minivacation. It's hard to think about your problems if you're lost in a captivating thriller, romance, or comedy. It's hard to think about yourself while reading unless your mind wanders, and if it does, it may not be a very good book.

HUMOR

One of the most important techniques for being good to yourself is humor. Find ways to incorporate humor and joy into your life. Dr. Steve Allen, Jr., a physician who is also a motivational speaker, advises people to "see the irony in your situation, and use it to fuel your humor. Know that humor is okay. There is great health in humor. It's a healthy response to tragedy, a language to express our emotions.

"Don't be so self-conscious about humor. Try to add humor to your life, but if your jokes don't make anyone laugh, it's not a terrible thing. At least you tried. You don't need to get X amount of silliness in each day."

Dr. Norman Decker stresses another benefit of humor: "A couple I've worked with for a number of months had argued for years about a certain issue. Once they introduced some humor into the issue, it reduced the overwhelming emotional aspect of it. Humor improved their sense of connection with each other. Once they could joke about it, they felt close. The issue was no longer something between them, no longer an obstacle."

HOPE

Finally, never give up hope. "Without hope for something, life—even if it's short—becomes oppressive," advises Dr. Decker. "But if you hope for something, it makes what remains of your lives together worthwhile."

If you hope for something unrealistic, then you won't be prepared when problems arise. You may even be emotionally traumatized.

You might hope that your situation or the skills you learn will enable you to help or teach others. You might hope to become a more sensitive person and to understand life better, or to share your experiences by writing about them or volunteering to speak about them.

Families often have hopes that, even if a relative dies, they will stick together; that they will overcome past arguments; that someone will be with their loved one if he is scared at night. And many people hope they can discover new things to laugh at and enjoy.

Rabbi Samuel E. Karff, senior rabbi of Congregation Beth Israel in Houston, suggests that there are three tracks to hope besides focusing on a cure. "The first is that you will be able to handle whatever you must cope with. The second is that the patient will live long enough to fulfill his responsibilities to those who need him. The third is religious—you hope God will be there with you and your loved ones."

Whether you wish for the world to change dramatically or for a peaceful evening with the patient, having a realistic hope can be the cornerstone to your well-being.

You won't be able to use all the techniques, guidelines, and suggestions in this chapter. I hope, however, that you'll incorporate some of them into your life. Because what is most precious is you. You are as important as everyone else in your life. Taking care of yourself will ensure that you can take care of those you love.

Besides yourself and the patient, the most important people you have to take care of are your children. In the next two chapters I'll show you ways to help them cope when a loved one has cancer.

Chapter 9

Sharing the News and Helping Children Understand When a Loved One Is Ill

Anna was the kind of girl people notice. Her huge, trusting brown eyes were almost as striking as her waist-length tendrils of twisting hair. Her fifteen-year-old wit charmed everyone. But no one appreciated her as Jeremy did. He adored his daughter. Yet when he got cancer, the laughter, the talking, and the long evenings they had spent together came to an end.

He never told her why his eyes were now surrounded by sunken lines, or why his bones protruded from his emaciated arms, or why he spent not only his nights but many of his days curled beneath the covers, behind closed doors. She did not understand why he withdrew. Instead, she imagined she had done something wrong; therefore, he no longer wanted her.

Looking back, Anna's mother, Nancy, pondered her role in what happened. "I suppose I should have told Anna about her father, but I was so caught up in my own grief, my own shock, I couldn't talk to anyone about this disease, especially her."

Jeremy recovered. Anna did not. After two years of vigorous treatments, the cancer was gone. Anna was pregnant, drinking heavily and sneaking out her bedroom window at night. Sometimes she'd leave for days, sometimes for weeks. After giving birth to Tim, Anna climbed out that window one last time, leaving her son behind for her parents to raise.

She never wrote. She never called. Through friends and relatives, Nancy and Jeremy knew where she was and what she was doing. But against their deepest desires, they did not go to talk to her. They sent short messages, notes, and presents, all by way of the relatives. But Anna did not respond. "There were times when we had to see her," Jeremy remembered. "We'd drive to this parking lot, across the street from where she worked. We'd sit for hours waiting for her to emerge from her job as a waitress, just to catch a moment's glance, a sideways look, anything. Then she'd get into her car and was gone again."

Fifteen years later, Jeremy's cancer returned. Until then, Tim had been "a good boy," said Nancy, "never a bit of trouble. A football player with above-average grades. And he had such nice friends."

Two months into Jeremy's chemotherapy, however, Tim started climbing out the same window Anna had. His grades dropped. The nice friends disappeared. Nancy discovered drugs in his room. Still, she and Jeremy thought they could handle Tim. Until he almost died of an overdose.

Jeremy and Nancy decided they weren't going to lose another child. They joined my weekly support group for couples coping with cancer. Two months after they finished the group, Nancy wrote me a letter. "Tim is getting all A's and B's. He's drug-free. After following your advice, we sent letters to Anna, sharing the feelings we never knew how to share before."

She continued, "We are better parents now, and closer as a couple. You have helped us to prevent the past from repeating itself. We can't change what happened with Anna, but we have changed the way we raise Tim.

"Then last week as I was fixing dinner, someone knocked at our door. No one ever visits us unannounced. I expected to see a person who had lost his way.

"There she stood, twisting a tendril of her dark wavy hair, those piercing eyes smiling up at me. I pulled Anna in and cried, tears I never knew I had, tears I had kept locked away all those years. As I held her, wanting never to let her go again, I could see Tim. Without a word, he leaped toward the door, scooped us off our feet, encircling Anna and me in his huge arms.

"As I write this, I can hear Anna, Jeremy, and Tim laughing in the other room. I know all too well what pain this disease brings, but you showed us how we could turn our tragedy into an opportunity to bring our daughter home."

The advice Jeremy and Nancy used to help themselves is included throughout this book. The guidelines they followed for their daughter and grandson are included in the next two chapters. They will help you support your children when someone important in their lives is ill, be it a parent, schoolteacher, grandparent, aunt, or friend of the family. The closer the relationship, the harder it will hit them. Although I use only parents with cancer as examples here, the guidelines can be adapted to any adult. You may not be able to use all of these suggestions, but read through them and decide which ones you can use.

When a significant person in a child's life is ill, the child will be confronted with issues and questions, many of which she may not be able to articulate. Nevertheless, children are more perceptive than we think. Children as young as four years old have explained aspects of this disease quite accurately. Don't underestimate your child's ability to understand. By learning as much as you can about how children react to this situation, you will be able to help your child understand, adjust to, and even grow from the catastrophic illness that is about to disrupt his entire life.

Every family has a unique set of values, beliefs, and circumstances. How *you* approach this illness will depend on these factors:

Whether anyone close to you has a similar disease
The ages of your children
Where you live—the culture of the neighborhood, be it in a large city or small town
Whether this is a first or second marriage
The presence of extended family members, friends, or congregation members who will help your family
A history of family illness
The birth of a child
A recent move or any other major life change
How you deal with illness

These factors will also contribute to how *your* family handles the illness.

Although your first instinct may be to protect your children from bad news, keeping information from them will cause even more problems than informing them will. Children may not know exactly what is wrong, but they will sense that something bad has happened. They are extremely sensitive to alterations in their parents' moods and changes in their environments. And the diagnosis will create changes in all of your lives. Telling your children sets the tone for how these changes will be made. Explaining this disease is going to be one of the hardest things you have ever had to do. Your children's reactions to it may upset you. They may storm out of the room crying, or they may act as if they do not care. Regardless of their behavior, you can provide them with guidance to cope with the coming challenges.

After you tell them, you may not know what your kids want or what they are feeling. I know it seems hard to believe now, but in the weeks and months to come, you will learn how to talk to them and how to understand their needs. And they may surprise you. Children who learn to communicate openly and share with their parents grow closer to them. Relationships become stronger, and a deeper love for each other develops. I've talked to children five, six, and ten years after they had been in Cancer Counseling's program. As a result of their experiences, they were more understanding and compassionate. They were proud of the social and coping skills they had developed—skills that you can teach your children. But before we look at those skills, you must confront the hardest job you will ever have: giving them the news.

Before You Tell Them

1. Evaluate your own feelings about the illness.

The hardest part about talking with your children is tolerating your own feelings while you tell them. No matter how you tell them or how they react, you will still hurt for them. The more comfortable you are with your emotions, the easier it will be to tell them. One way to reduce some of the pain is to learn more about helping them. The more equipped you feel to support them, the less pain you will all experience.

2. Read and find out as much as you can.

- Call a social service agency and ask to speak to a counselor. Even if the agency is not in your area, they will often provide telephone support. Expert help is worth the long-distance phone bill.
- Ask a social worker at the hospital where the patient is being treated if you can meet with him to discuss your children.
- A school counselor may have experience working with children of cancer patients, or else she may be able to refer you to a qualified therapist.
- Ask your librarian or a bookstore employee to recommend books, tapes, and other teaching tools that explain illness or the life cycle in age-appropriate terms.
- Attend a free support group. If you aren't comfortable talking to strangers, ask if you can just observe the meeting to get ideas.

3. You can tell children of different ages separately or together. Regardless, set time aside afterward to talk to each child individually.

Children of different ages and maturity will react to the news according to where they are developmentally. A four-year-old views the world from one perspective, a six-year-old from another.

One of my staff members brought a family into her office and plopped the five-year-old onto her lap, while the six-year-old held Daddy's hand and the teenager sat between her parents. Together they talked about the cancer.

Afterward, the counselor saw the children individually. The youngest child's questions were focused on losing Mommy, even though the prognosis was good. The six-year-old was angry: "This is all Daddy's fault. He didn't take care of Mommy." The teenager withdrew, not wanting to share her feelings at all.

Reggie, another five-year-old, had parents who discussed the disease in family meetings. This was fine, except that they never spoke to their children separately. Consequently, their two younger children, who were uncomfortable asking questions in front of the big kids, did not fully understand as much as they could have if the parents had talked to them individually.

When I interviewed Reggie, her mother had taken a turn for the worse and was receiving support from hospice services. The father told me he thought Reggie had absolutely no understanding that her mother was dying. While he waited in another office, Reggie told me that Mommy was very sick and was going to heaven forever, with Reggie's aunt, who used to live in the backyard. Reggie added, "But it's okay. My aunt needs my mom more than we do. And besides, I'll see her in heaven soon."

When I asked her father to clarify, he told me that Reggie's aunt had indeed lived in the backyard. Well, not quite—her house had been directly behind theirs. The aunt had recently died. What Reggie didn't understand was that her mommy and aunt were going to be gone forever. She believed that heaven was a place that she could visit very soon. A child's concept of time is completely different from an adult's. At Reggie's age, forever is an abstract idea, difficult to understand.

Young children will sense something is wrong and feel bad about what you will tell them. Yet they won't have the vocabulary or the developmental skills to articulate what they are feeling. They may repeat back what you say, while understanding only parts of it. They may also react by clinging or acting out their feelings while playing. Watch how young children play. Their fantasy worlds will give you clues as to how they will deal with this ordeal. Their make-believe, magical stories will include scenarios related to the ill parent. The stories may have superheroes—most likely themselves—who have these magical powers and can make the parent better or worse. Creating fantasies is children's way of dealing with their fears and anxieties. It is developmentally appropriate and can be a good way for them to express their emotions. Unfortunately, magical thinking can lead to children taking undue responsibility for the disease if it is not explained to them. They may believe they caused the cancer. The world, after all, revolves around them, so they must be responsible for any problems in it.

Children who are Reggie's age may also seem confused or embarrassed by conversations about illness. They may laugh, giggle, or change the subject. Or they may seem to accept the news like little troupers but have only a vague notion about certain aspects of it, as Reggie did. To her, Mommy's condition was sad but wouldn't last forever.

For teenagers and young adolescents, the normal developmental stage is to begin their independence, to break away from their parents and establish their own identities. It is a tough time, a period when peer support and acceptance is vital to their identity. They want to be like everybody else, and they are concerned and sometimes obsessed with getting involved with members of the opposite sex, finding and developing their first loves. The news of a parent's illness affects them in several ways. It draws them back into the home, making the process of separation confusing. They may feel guilty or resentful, or they may abandon normal activities altogether, such as sports or being with their peers. Teenagers can struggle with internal as well as external battles.

Grace joined one of my bereavement groups a few weeks after her fifty-one-year-old husband died. Throughout the first session, she couldn't stop crying, ripping Kleenex after Kleenex from the box beside her and squirming in her chair. For two years she had endured her daughter's attacks. "Emily has an endless reservoir of cruel comments," she said, "all of which she directs at me."

The father, as we later learned from Emily, was too ill to be a target: "I couldn't yell at Daddy. He needed me."

It took several weeks for Grace to reach a place in her own grief before she was ready to address her daughter's: "I am well aware that it is grief and fear and confusion that led to Emily's behavior, but understanding her isn't enough. I need to know how to talk to her. Throughout this entire ordeal I have had no idea what to say."

It wasn't too late. The techniques in this chapter and the next taught her how to help Emily talk about her feelings. Once Emily was able to express herself and accept her mother's love, they began to rebuild their fractured relationship.

An illness can disrupt childhood development by pushing a child too quickly ahead or by leaving him stranded and confused. After you have told your children, regardless of their age they will need your individual support to work through these complex issues. Although Emily's problems were ultimately resolved, many of them could have been avoided. If Grace had known how to talk to Emily, the walls separating her from her daughter would never have been erected. I can't promise you that using these guidelines will ensure that your child won't act like Emily, but you will have more knowledge and information than Grace had. That alone will enable you to help your children in ways she couldn't.

Telling Your Children

4. Ask them what they already know about the disease.

Most children have heard about cancer and other serious illnesses. Ask younger children: "What does the word *cancer* mean to you? Do you know anyone with cancer? What happened? How does someone get cancer? Have you seen a cancer patient on television? Do you remember the movie we saw where someone had it? What do you think happens when a person gets cancer?" Ask them if they remember a relative or neighbor who is now in remission: "Do you remember when Uncle So-and-So was sick?"

These questions can help you assess where your children are before you share the news with them. Ask teenagers similar questions, to learn what their experiences are. They may have a better understanding of the disease. Yet they may have been exposed only to patients who were dying and therefore assume that everyone dies of cancer. On the other hand, they may know only of people who recovered. If that does not appear to be the prognosis, explain to them what the doctors have told you. Ways to clarify this are in this chapter and the next.

5. Be honest, upbeat, and realistic.

Kids can handle even the worst news surprisingly well, if you tell it to them in ways they can comprehend. But if you don't tell them what is happening, they may imagine the situation is worse than it is. They may think the patient is dying, for example, when in fact he is experiencing only the temporary side effects of chemotherapy. Misinformation is often more frightening and confusing to children than the truth.

Obviously, the worst news is that a parent is dying. It needs to be discussed with children in depth. They may think that if Daddy dies or leaves them, Mommy will leave too, or they may believe they will catch the disease and die. You can explain the essential facts without sharing every gory detail.

No matter what happens, be realistic. If the patient has only weeks to live or months of treatment to undergo, do not tell your kids,

"Everything will be fine very soon." Now is the time to prepare them for what lies ahead. Your honesty will set the groundwork for the type of relationship you will have with them for the rest of your lives.

Try to give them as accurate a timetable as possible about the length of the treatment: "The doctors hope Daddy will complete treatment by Halloween," you might say. Or: "Daddy should be home from the hospital by next weekend."

In language your child can understand, tell him what disease the parent has and what is going to be done about it. Use real terms and correct information. Social worker Priscilla L. Hartung, director of social services at Cancer Care in New York City, advises, "When telling younger children, keep it simple and to the point. Say, 'One cell got out of control, and we have to take medicine to try to control it.'"

Dr. Brendan O'Rourke, a child psychologist with Cancer Counseling, adds, "It's difficult with younger children. Under the age of twelve, children don't think abstractly. Try to use examples that are concrete to some extent. With children ages five to eight, say, 'Mommy has cancer. Mommy is real sick. There are bad cells that aren't supposed to be in her body. They are fighting the good cells. When the bad cells are winning, it makes her sick. We are going to do surgery or give her medicine to try to get rid of the bad cells. We don't know for sure why this happened.'

"If they ask if they can get the cancer, say, 'Sometimes children do get cancer, but it is very rare. If you ever have concerns, we can talk to your pediatrician.'"

Other examples of what you might say:

> "The doctor is going to make Mommy comfortable
> for as long as he can."
> "These pills [show them the medication] will help
> make Daddy better. The medicine is very strong,
> and it might make him sick. But when he gets sick,
> it doesn't mean he is getting worse or he is going
> to die. We are trying to kill the bad cells, but the

medicine can make the good cells upset for a little while."

"We can't be sure about what will happen, but we will tell you how she is doing as we go along."

Dr. O'Rourke advises that "it's important to balance honesty with reassurance. It's like a dance. You don't want to go too far in either direction. Never be brutally honest, because children hang on to vivid language. If you are going to use vivid language, use it about positive things, not negative ones."

Children ages eight to eleven may have other concerns that you should be prepared to handle. Excerpts from eight-year-old Michael Kim's diary give insights into what your child may be thinking. Michael's father had stopped working and was on chemotherapy when Michael wrote, "I worry about money."

Michael's mother, Lucy, said, "Thank goodness he showed me that diary. I was able to reassure him that financially things were tight but that we would work them out. It was amazing how an eight-year-old concluded that since Daddy didn't get up and go to work as he used to, we would have problems with money. Where were we going to get food and clothes? he worried. Where was the money coming from?"

Michael's next excerpt brought up another concern: "I worry about my dad while I'm at school." Explains Lucy, "Because his dad was very sick after the chemotherapy treatments, Michael didn't know what he would find when he came home. When he read this passage to me, I realized I had to keep him informed about everything we were doing. I would prepare him before we went to the hospital to get chemotherapy. I told him more about what each day might be like, because if I didn't, he would think it would be worse than it was. The truth was always easier than what he imagined."

The hardest excerpt for Lucy to deal with was the one where he wrote, "I wish my dad would talk more." Lucy explains, "His dad didn't feel well a lot and wasn't able to do things with him. But to a child that was personal. I told Michael, 'It's not because your dad doesn't want to talk to you. It's that he doesn't feel well.' "

And the last excerpt was "I wish my dad would eat dinner with me." Again, Lucy explains that "dinner had been a family ritual. Because his dad had trouble eating, he couldn't join us anymore. The ritual fell apart. There were a lot of rituals like that. I had to explain why he couldn't eat with us, then come up with new rituals. Children thrive on rituals, and though they may not be able to verbalize why they mean so much, they notice when rituals aren't followed."

Taking your children to visit the patient's doctor may help address other concerns that they may not be verbalizing, such as "Where is Mommy going today?" "What's it like at that office?" A visit will correct any misinformation they may have acquired or imagined.

Dr. Ernest Katz explains how to inform young adolescents and teenagers: "The important thing is for the parents to provide truthful information, emphasizing hopefulness. Explain what this means in terms of the treatment the patient will be going through and how it will affect the family. Tell them, 'There are things we can do. We are hopeful.' Even if the parent is going to die, hope for a good quality of life can still be maintained.

"Teenagers will fluctuate back and forth. They may feel bad, guilty, or angry at the disruption in their lives, asking, 'Why does this have to happen now?' "

Whether your teenagers will ask questions about the illness depends on their personality. "Some children are quite able," Dr. Katz adds. "But many may be embarrassed or afraid to upset the parents. So I suggest including teenagers on one of the regular medical visits. This will give them an opportunity to meet with a sympathetic physician or someone else on the patient's health care team. The visit can be arranged beforehand. Call the office or the hospital, and ask if a member of the medical team has experience and is sympathetic to speaking with teenagers. The professional could just take a few minutes to walk with a child down the hall for a Coke. During this meeting the teenager could express her feelings and ask questions. This way her questions will be dealt with directly."

6. Teach your children how to hope for things other than a cure.

No matter what the prognosis may be, let your children know this disease is very serious and that no one can predict its outcome. Help your children understand the importance of hoping for the best even if you have to prepare for the worst. If you paint a picture in which nothing can go wrong, they will have a difficult time if complications arise. Explain how you are hoping for the very best but that no one can guarantee positive results.

One way to do this is to teach your children to hope for other things besides a cure. Focus on each day's positive events. Work with them to create meaningful ways to spend time with the patient: playing board games with him, looking at family albums, or doing homework together. Give the child ways to help the patient, such as by bringing a blanket, finding a video he wants, preparing a special meal, or telling the parent about school activities.

Even if the prognosis is poor, there are positive goals you can help your children hope to achieve—to share an upcoming holiday, to go to the movies that weekend, to watch a favorite movie or sports event together, to read a book before bed at night, or to plan a special evening.

A cure and a long life are not the only things children can be taught to hope for. Short-term plans and precious moments are important too.

7. Tell children cancer is not caused by a person or by an event like a divorce.

A forty-year-old engineer who had cancer proudly announced to me that he knew he was going to be cured: "I know what caused this—my ex-wife. Now that I'm divorced, I will be able to get rid of the cancer." This man had part-time custody of his children. Can you imagine if he talked this way around them? If he did, they would learn that Mommy or a bad relationship can cause cancer. A divorce can cure it.

Another man in my program had in fact won a lawsuit against a chemical company where he worked, claiming the chemicals caused his cancer. He told his fourteen-year-old son about the lawsuit. His son decided, "I'm never going to work, because that's how my daddy got sick."

Assure your children that the cancer is no one's fault. Don't ever say, "Well, your daddy worked too hard, and that's why he got cancer." Or: "Your mom was under a lot of stress, so now she's sick." If they ask about smoking, it is more complicated. You need to say, "Smoking is bad, and it may have caused Mommy's cancer"—but only if the doctor has said that the cell type of the cancer shows it is the kind associated with smoking. However, blaming the patient achieves nothing. The focus has to be on handling *what* has happened, not on *why* it happened.

You will never know exactly what caused your loved one's cancer, so you won't be able to give your kids an accurate explanation. Why does one person who smokes get cancer while another does not? The causes of this disease are so complicated that even the most qualified experts will rarely pinpoint a specific cause. Do everything you can to convince your kids not to smoke, but try to find other reasons besides a parent's lung cancer. This is one question you ought to answer, "I don't know what made Daddy sick, except for the bad cells."

As I mentioned earlier, younger children may be afraid that they caused the disease, or they can make the disease better or worse. They believe certain acts cause other, unrelated acts. "I left my toy in the room, and Mommy fell over it, and then she had cancer." "I haven't been good in school, and now her cancer is worse." "I yelled at Mom, and that's why she's sicker." "I made her cry, and it made the side effects worse."

Explain to your children that doing something bad does not make the cancer worse, and doing something good doesn't make it better. Do not wait for your kids to verbalize these imaginings. Make it very clear from the outset that nothing they did or said has anything to do with the cancer.

8. *Explain why cancer is not contagious.*

Even some adults think they can "catch" cancer. No wonder, then, that children often fear they will catch it, or that the other parent will catch it. It is important to tell children of all ages that cancer is not something you can catch.

Explain why it's not like a cold, the flu, or the chicken pox. Patients can't give it to anyone else—nor can they catch it from anyone else.

9. *Be comfortable saying "I don't know."*

When you don't know the answer or you aren't comfortable with a question, admit, "I don't know the answer right now, but I'll let you know as soon as I do." Then research the question by talking to a child psychologist, a social worker, or your pediatrician. Seeking answers will also give you an opportunity to learn more.

Some questions can only be answered with time. Others may never have solutions. Help your children understand and accept these realities.

10. *While you are telling children about the disease, watch for signals indicating how they are taking it.*

If a child stiffens, dodges questions, looks away, raises his shoulders, or acts angry or defensive, be careful how much you share. He may not be ready to hear any more at this time.

If necessary, separate the children and tell them individually as much as each seems able to handle. You don't have to bombard them with a long dissertation the first time you tell them. They need to assimilate the news at their own pace. It's okay if it takes several discussions spaced out over time to tell them all the details. When they start asking you questions in the course of a normal day, you will know that they are ready to hear more. If they do not ask additional questions, it will be up to you to initiate the next discussion.

11. Each child reacts in her own way, and even the same child can have many different reactions to the news.

One child may be stoic. Another cries. Another will try to comfort you. Another will get angry. And the same child may be calm one day and angry the next. Children don't always react in ways we would expect. They need you to understand their reactions no matter what they are. However they react is the "normal" way for them to handle the news.

12. It's okay to cry.

Your tears give them permission to cry, either alone or with you. You can say, "Your mommy's illness makes me very sad. It's okay to cry when you are sad." Or: "You may feel sad too." They will learn that crying is a normal reaction.

If they cry and you don't, validate their emotions: "I felt that way too when I heard." Or: "There are times when I cry too because Daddy is ill."

13. Let them know that there will always be someone to take care of them.

During a support group, a wife of a patient shared her daughters' fears: "My girls asked, 'Who will take care of us if Daddy dies?' I said I would. Then they asked, 'What if something happens to you?' I had to go through a whole list of relatives before they felt they would not be abandoned."

14. Be prepared for anger.

Children can be mad at getting less attention, mad at the cancer, or mad at the parent for getting sick. They may pick more fights with each other. They may get more irritable or act out in passive-aggressive ways. Their anger can be a way of saying, "I feel helpless," "I'm here too," "You don't care about me," or "I'm scared." An angry outburst may be an opening for you to comment, "I wonder if you are mad because Mommy is sick."

Social worker Priscilla L. Hartung advises parents to acknowledge the anger by saying, "I'd be angry too," or "I'd be frightened too."

"With adolescents it's more complex," she goes on to explain. "You want to help them talk with their mouths instead of their fists. Yet you don't want to expose their emotions too quickly. If they realize that you're not afraid of them, that you only want to be supportive and to understand them, then you have made some inroads."

Dr. Donna Copeland, a clinical psychologist at M. D. Anderson Cancer Center, advises parents to "try to understand what the child is trying to get when he acts out. If he's anxious or upset, find constructive ways to channel his energy."

To help discharge the anger, you could say, "You may be very mad right now, but it's not okay to break your toys. Why don't you go outside and play [a sport they like]." Or: "I feel frustrated too. Let's go out and play some basketball together [or take a walk, or ride bikes]."

When the child has calmed down, ask her what motivated the anger. "Was something else bothering you yesterday? It's not like you to kick the cat."

In an article in the *St. Louis Post-Dispatch,* social worker Doris Wild Helmering suggests holding a family meeting to talk about the children's anger: "Ask your child for his cooperation in controlling his anger. Also, remind him that you expect him to control his anger at home just as he controls it at school.

"If you, the parent, have a problem with controlling your own anger, chances are your child will point this out at the family powwow. Decide that you too will work to control your anger.

"Invite your child to say over and over in his head during the day for the next several months, 'I choose not to get angry.' Repeating this affirmation reinforces the decision not to become angry.

"Suggest to your child that when he feels furious, instead of gritting his teeth and doing something mean, he should try to sing his favorite song in his head or repeat a favorite joke to himself. I told one little boy this, and he looked at me like I was nuts. But the next time I saw him, he couldn't wait to report that it had worked. A similar technique is to suggest to your child that when he feels himself getting angry, he should go to a chair, sit down, close his eyes, and see himself playing on the playground or swimming in a pool. This is called imaging. It helps the mind to calm the body and dissipate the adrenaline that accompanies angry feelings.

"Another technique is to ask your child not to allow himself to explode when he feels angry. When he feels anger coming on, tell him to purse his lips, set the timer on the stove for four minutes, and breathe deeply until the timer goes off. Once he's controlled himself for four minutes, he's won the battle.

"Ask your child to write down why he feels angry. Reassure him that within a half hour of putting pen to paper, you will read what he has written.

"Just as children need help learning to tie their shoes, write a report, iron a shirt, or throw a ball, they need help learning to control their anger. Take the time to give your children this skill, which will serve them the rest of their lives."

15. Learn how to talk about dying.

At some point, your children may ask you to explain death, even if the patient has a great prognosis. It's better to be prepared for this

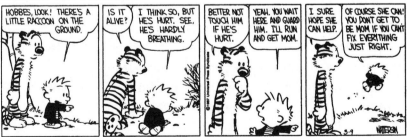

Calvin and Hobbes © 1987 Watterson. Dist. by Universal Press Syndicate. Reprinted with permission. All rights reserved.

question than to be thrown off guard by it. There are many ways to discuss death and dying. One is to discuss it in terms of your religious views. Another is to associate it with the life cycle.

"If the patient is terminal," Dr. O'Rourke advises, "say, 'From what the doctors tell us, it looks like the bad-guy cells are winning.' Or: 'We don't want them to win, but they might, and if at some point it looks like they are going to win, we are going to have to say good-bye. When one of your friends moves to another city, you give them something to keep, or you do something so they remember you. You might want to do that now. You could write a note or play Nintendo together, or you may want to give your father ten hugs or tell him how much you love him. This gives him something of yours to hold on to.'

"Let them know that the parent will not hurt anymore. If you want to discuss it in religious terms, say, 'He will be okay. He will be in heaven with God.' Reassure him that God is taking care of him. 'Everyone has their time to be with God. Sometimes when a person has been hurting or sick, God can take the pain away.'"

Some therapists warn that if you use heaven as an analogy for death, children may have problems with spirituality. They may be afraid that God is going to take them, or they may get mad at God for taking away the parent. They may think heaven is such a great place that, as Lucy Kim puts it, "Michael wanted to go there, and he did things to try to go there." However, as Dr. O'Rourke points out, "Heaven is a difficult concept to grasp. And children may not understand it completely, but you still have to talk in terms of what your family believes.

"Now, if you want to use the life cycle as an analogy, describe death in terms of the circle of life as it is shown in *The Lion King*. In the movie, Simba, the baby lion, carries on his father's hopes and dreams. A child's job is to keep the cycle going, to carry on the circle of life. They should remember the good things, take their parent's ideas and spirit into their minds and hearts. They should remember what the parent taught them. And tell them, 'We can find a little special place inside us to hold those memories. Sometimes we find something outside of us, like the stars, as Simba did. The stars remind us of the special gifts Daddy gave us.' "

When Simba looked up at the stars, he remembered his father and all he had taught him. Of the various ways to teach children about dying, watching this movie together may be one of the best.

However you explain it, do not ever say that the parent is going to sleep. Then the child may worry, "If Daddy went to sleep and never woke up, I might not either." This can cause night terrors, nightmares, and insomnia. Also be prepared to field practical questions. Here are two examples:

> Question: "Where is Daddy going to sleep?"
> Answer: "He will sleep in heaven" or "he doesn't need to sleep anymore."
> Question: "Where is Daddy going to eat?"
> Answer: "Daddy doesn't need to eat anymore."

From my work with teenagers, I've found that the best way to prepare them is to explain dying in a straightforward, honest manner. Do not try to be a cheerleader or encourage them to feel a certain way. Instead, let them know you are there to talk about their fears, their concerns, and whatever else they want to discuss. Acknowledge and validate their emotions, and let them know you don't want them to handle this crisis alone, that you want to go through it with them. Go to the movies together, and on the way home ask how they felt about a character who died or overcame an obstacle. They may not be able to talk directly about their ill parent, but they may be able to talk about a character they saw in a movie.

Whenever you are discussing dying, don't end the conversation without helping the child focus on what he can do today with the ill parent. Say, "Mommy is here now, and there are still lots of ways you can be together. No matter what happens, Mommy will always love you, and you will always love her. You can carry Mommy in your heart forever."

When I think of my son who died, I picture his ashes in the rose garden, but I also think about how close he is to me, how I carry his spirit in my heart. I think of a note Lucy sent me: "Now you have your own guardian angel." These kinds of thoughts are comforting for people of all ages.

16. Do not whisper.

Be careful not to whisper to anyone about the person who is ill when a child could be listening in. Include children in conversations about the disease or don't speak about it when they can hear only bits and pieces. Respect them. You wouldn't whisper in front of your friends or your spouse.

17. Children grieve too.

Children, like adults, grieve. When their parent's health is threatened, they are going to grieve many losses. If you tell them, "Don't cry, be strong," most likely they will only suppress their emotions, or exhibit them in other ways—by getting poor grades, withdrawing, or acting as though everything is fine.

Allowing them to cry can release the pain. When they stop crying, say, "I love you. I'm sorry this is so hard on you. I'm always here for you, and we're going to get through this together."

18. Ask children if they have understood what you said.

Young children may interpret your words to have different meanings from what you intended. Older kids may hear your optimism and interpret it to mean "Mommy will be cured."

If a parent is going to undergo treatment for months or years, explain the situation. Otherwise your children may think, as the treatment continues, "Daddy must be sicker than you're telling me. You just don't want me to know." Or: "He's going to die." Or: "You don't really think the treatment will work."

19. Keep children updated.

Once your children know the diagnosis and the preliminary treatment plan, keep them informed about any changes in the patient's medical status. Whatever you do, don't lie to them. Cancer is often a long illness—a marathon, not a sprint. It may be months or even years before the treatment ends. Any lie you tell now will affect your relationship with your children later. The best approach is to continually update them with accurate and pertinent information, including any expectations about how long treatment will last.

20. Make only promises you can keep.

You want to ease the pain your children are feeling. So you may make promises to them and *hope you can keep them*. Such promises may make you and your children feel better for the moment. But they are going to experience many disappointments as a result of the patient's illness. Unkept promises will just add to those disappointments—if not today, then in the future. If you are fairly confident you can fulfill the promise, however, you can say, "I will try..."

21. Reassure children of your love.

They need your unconditional love. Sometimes you may not like their behavior, but you always love them. Moreover, they need reassurance of your love on a continual basis. It can be the security blanket they hang on to through the weeks and months ahead.

You may think you have told them everything they need to know. You assume they understood you. They may have understood at that time, but a few days later, they may have questions that show they do not. Tell them:

"I've just given you a lot of new information. It's going to take a while to digest it all. So please come back when you've thought about it, and we can talk some more."

"Sometimes things are very hard to understand, or confusing, or scary. You don't have to figure it out all at once, but I will be here to help you, and we will try to figure this out together. Please let's keep talking about this. It takes a while to understand."

And how do you keep "talking about it"? How do you encourage and empower them to handle their greatest challenge, living with a loved one's illness? The next chapter will give you ways to guide your children through this very long journey—a journey that will, regardless of the outcome, affect them for the rest of their lives.

Chapter 10

A Family Challenge:
Overcoming the Long-Term Problems

Dr. Ernest Katz works with children whose parents have cancer. I asked him if he followed up on any of them afterward. He said, "There was a young man I worked with when he was twelve. His mother died of cancer, and his father had a hard emotional time dealing with the loss of his wife. There were two kids. The older sister rapidly moved out after the death, which left the twelve-year-old to try to hold his father together. It was an incredible burden for this young man. Fortunately, we finally got his father into counseling. His son became extremely compassionate as a result of his experience. He started volunteering with kids with cancer, working with summer camps."

"So what happened to him?" I asked.

"He's in medical school. He's going to be a doctor," Dr. Katz responded.

"Any other stories?" I asked.

He thought for a moment. "Yes, mine. I was fifteen when my

mother had cancer. In the mid-sixties no one was talking about cancer, not even within families. My father would come into my room in the middle of the night and whisper to me about my mother. Up until the time my mother died, she and I never talked about it. That was more than twenty years ago, yet I am still processing that whole experience. I'm a clinical psychologist. My life's work has always been focused on children because I feel kids aren't listened to."

As a teenager, I myself watched both a friend and my grandfather suffer from this disease. You are reading this book because of what I did with the pain of my friend's death and my grandfather's illness.

Not all children who have had a similar experience go into the helping professions. One young boy took part in Cancer Counseling's program when he was twelve years old and four feet tall. At eighteen he returned to participate in a documentary, all six feet of him. Towering over me, he was one of the sweetest kids I had met in years. "I just want to help in any way I can," he said. When he was twenty-two, he started his own computer business. He was quite the little entrepreneur. The last I heard, the business was thriving. The name he used for his business was his father's, a man who can be found on most afternoons leaning over all sorts of gadgets, pointing at his son, asking, "This is where these go. Are you following me?"

After you tell your children the news, you may think nothing good could ever come of such a horrific experience. The road that lies ahead is surely going to be difficult, but it does hold many gifts. You have the opportunity and the power to teach your children to turn tragedy into triumph. You can enable them to adapt to the disruptions in their lives. You can facilitate their ability to learn new skills, to acquire new strengths, and to grow from this experience. In fact, your children may learn skills that most people never learn: compassion, patience, hope, understanding, and most important, love.

Sometimes we gain our greatest strengths through adversity. I know I have. Adversity makes us work that much harder to perfect whatever it is we have set out to learn. The guidelines in this chapter will give you ways to help your children explore their feelings. They will also give you practical techniques to use when faced with difficult decisions. You will be amazed at how incorporating these ideas into your life can empower your children.

Helping Children Understand and Integrate Their Feelings

1. Create ways to express feelings.

More often than not, the moments your child is ready to talk about her feelings are those you are least prepared for. You can, however, create an environment that encourages the expression of her feelings.

As Dr. Mitch Golant, vice president of the Wellness Community National and co-author of *The Challenging Child,* says, "The world is full of teachable moments. Sometimes you have to follow your children's clues." Other times you have to create those moments yourself. Here are ways to create opportunities for children to express their emotions. Decide which will work best with your children.

Storytelling and Playing

This is a good way to help younger children understand their feelings. Use a doll or toy, and start the story with, "When Big Bird didn't feel well, he went to the doctor and found out he had cancer." Tell the story yourself, or have your children join in. They can describe how Big Bird got to the doctor and handled the news, then how he took the medications and how he acted afterward.

Encourage them to write a short story or poem about when the parent got sick. They can write a letter to her telling her their feelings. They can write a letter to a friend or relative, sharing stories about the changes in their lives.

Validate their emotions by sharing with them an experience that happened to you. "I remember when my father had cancer. I was very scared." They'll then know it's okay to be scared, mad, or sad, because you felt that way. Say, "When something like this happens, it's okay to feel..." Instead of "How are you feeling about Mommy's illness?" you could say, "Isn't it awful seeing someone you care about so sick?" Or: "It must be frustrating not to be able to have Mommy do the things she used to do with you." You can acknowledge their wish that the disease would disappear and their lives would return to normal: "I bet you wish this wasn't happening."

Watch an inspiring movie together about someone who has triumphed over a disease. Depending upon your loved one's prognosis, you may also choose a movie where someone dies—if he had an inspirational life up until the end. When the movie is over, talk about it. How did your children feel about the main character, the doctors, the hospital, the family members, the friends, and the disease? Your local video store manager may be able to recommend movies that would be good to use for children of different ages.

Another way to help children express their feelings is to bring up an article and show it to your child: "I read about a girl whose mother has cancer. She really had a hard time...."

If your child plays with dolls or any other toys that could represent feelings, use them to act out what is happening in the family. While children are busy playing house, or playing with Barney, the Muppets, Ninja Turtles, or stuffed animals, they may reveal their feelings. Playing games gives them an opportunity to express their reactions in a safe place. And their reactions may surprise you. Try to be comfortable with their emotions when they are playing. This is an easy way for them to discharge feelings.

Drawing
Drawing is another good technique for expressing emotions. Ask your children if they would like to draw pictures of the family. Have them explain what they are drawing while they are drawing it or after they have finished.

You can also use pictures to help children express their feelings. Try the following exercise at home with younger children.

Bring one child into a comfortable room—maybe the den or play-room. Sit with him, symbolizing that you're engaged in this exercise too. Have ready a chart with drawings of faces, each of which depicts a different emotion: anger, sadness, happiness, or nervousness. Cuddle up together (if it's comfortable for you) to establish some in-timacy. Then point to a face that represents how you feel. Ask your child, "Which of these drawings looks like how you feel?"

This exercise will give him a way to assign pictures to his feelings. Younger children don't analyze their feelings, so you need to help them by putting words or pictures to them. To help them verbalize, you can say, "You look so sad. It must feel like all of my attention is on Daddy now." A child who may think it's childish to be afraid of losing a parent or being abandoned may point to the sad face and share her fears.

Your children may feel more comfortable exposing their emotions this way than in a heart-to-heart talk. You could also draw faces or ask your child to draw her face. Then talk about the drawing. Get a set of children's magazines and together cut out pictures of different emotions. Help your kids use them to make up their own charts.

At Cancer Counseling I asked children to draw their home and the people in it, or to draw their family at the dinner table. As they drew very intricate, revealing portraits of their worlds, they often felt free to describe them.

Reading Together

Reading together is another activity that can foster the expression of feelings. Therapists recommend the following books. You may want to review them at the library to decide which may be most helpful for your children:

- *Sammy's Mommy Has Cancer,* Sherry Kohlenberg (Magination Press, 1993). This picture book includes information on Mommy being ill, losing her hair, and going to the hospital. For ages 2–6.

- *Gran-Gran's Best Trick,* Dwight Holden (Magination Press, 1989). This story is told from a young girl's point of view about her ill grandfather. For ages 4–9.
- *Gentle Willow,* Joyce Mills (Magination Press, 1983). The book uses a butterfly as a metaphor about living and dying.
- *Grandad Bill's Song,* Jane Yolen (Philomel Books, 1994). This book explores a child's feelings about his grandfather's death.
- *The Barn,* Avi (Orchid, 1994). A child confronts his fear and sadness about losing his father.

Since new books are always being published, call your librarian, your child's teacher, a professional counselor, or your bookstore. Ask what books they would recommend to help children understand their feelings. Parenting magazines (*Child, Parents,* and *American Baby*) list and sometimes review newly released books. Ask your librarian for the spring edition of *Publishers Weekly,* which has reviews of upcoming children's books. A book doesn't have to be only about illness to be helpful. Your children can learn about their feelings from many different kinds of stories, such as *The Lion King.* Any good story that teaches children about handling problems or a loss, or any story about the circle of life, may be of help.

Time Alone

Encourage your children to take time alone to evaluate and express their feelings. Suggest that they keep a journal. One of my clients bought notebooks for her two girls, ages seven and ten, and asked them if they'd like to write down what happened each day. The journals were a wonderful vehicle for the mother to start conversations about the girls' feelings. Even if the contents had never been discussed, the girls still would have treasured them for many years afterward. One of the girls wrote only a few times a month, while the other put down her feelings every night. The mother told me, "Neither girl could talk about her dad's illness, and he had been sick for almost a year. Once they wrote about their feelings, though, it opened up the floodgates.

After only two nights of writing, my younger daughter came to me and wanted to talk about her daddy. From that point on, she was comfortable discussing her worries, her hopes, and she no longer had a problem asking us questions."

2. Let your children set the pace.

When you are reading, playing, or drawing, let your children set the pace. They don't always have to finish a project. Let them engage in it for as long as they are interested. A child may write only a few lines in a journal, as Lucy Kim's children did. "Those few lines sparked their emotions and opened up the lines of communication," Lucy says. "It took only one week for it to work."

These ideas are to be used when you need that spark, a vehicle to start the conversation. Reading together may help bring out their feelings, but sometimes that won't work and you may want to try watching a movie together. Your child may want to see movies like *The Lion King* many times. Others he won't even want to sit through once. Let him lead you in these activities. You want him to share his emotions, but you also want it to be an enjoyable process.

3. Don't push them to talk about feelings.

You can't sit your child down in a chair and force him to have a heart-to-heart talk. It just won't work.

We've all had moments with children when we could almost see them grab hold of an invisible zipper and close it tightly around their mouths. We've seen, or given as children ourselves, *that look*. It says, "I don't have anything to say to you," or "You're an idiot," or "You don't understand."

A hug or a touch, or curling up and watching TV together, can allow children to feel close. They will bring up their feelings when they are ready. If not, there are other ways you can help them express feelings.

4. Pay attention to the indirect ways children bring up their concerns.

Children don't feel like you are scrutinizing them if you are busy doing routine things together. You may be driving, cleaning the kitchen, making a bed, or taking care of a pet, when your child brings up a movie he saw, a friend's ill parent, a teacher who talked about someone with cancer, or a pet that is ill.

The sick raccoon someone found at school can become a springboard for your conversation. All you may talk about is the raccoon. By discussing what happens to this animal, your child can explore your attitudes and her feelings about her parent's illness. You might ask, "Does the raccoon make you think about Daddy?"

Mood Swings and Danger Signs

5. Be ready for mood swings.

As children incorporate the changes in their lives, their emotions may become more volatile. Just as your moods can change from hour to hour and day to day, so can theirs. It is important that you address these changes by talking with your children as much as you can. If the changes become significant, seek support from a professional counselor.

6. Don't ignore changes in grades or in sleeping or eating patterns, or dramatic swings in behavior.

Your kids need extra care and understanding from you as they work through their feelings. Some kids act out because they don't have the verbal skills to express what they are feeling. Others have the verbal skills but are too confused to apply them.

They may be irritable or withdrawn, do poorly in school, act violently toward others, become hyperactive, or obsess about activities like sports. They may regress to a behavior they had outgrown, like bed-wetting or thumb-sucking.

If your child stops eating or sleeping, becomes violent, appears unusually depressed, or has any emotions that seem extreme to you or represent a significant change in behavior, then you should seek professional help. I believe that all families going through a catastrophic illness can benefit from counseling. Even if they only use it to prevent problems from occurring. But if your kids are already having problems, it's even more important to find a good professional. Their well-being is at stake. An expert can assess how serious the problems are and guide you and your children through the changes. (Sources for referrals can be found later in this chapter.)

If you think your children have handled the disease well and it hasn't *really* affected them, beware. Countless parents have told me how well their children are handling the changes that accompany a serious illness. Yet in most cases the children were actually protecting the parents. They either masked their problems in front of the parents, or else the parents didn't recognize the problems. Sometimes these problems are difficult to detect if the children's outward behavior is unchanged. In front of their parents, these kids smiled and were nonchalant. In my office they broke down in tears.

If you ask your children what they are feeling in a safe, nonjudgmental way, or follow some of the suggestions in this chapter, or take them to counseling, you will be able to uncover most of their concerns and learn how to address them positively.

Who Else Can Help?

7. Take your family to a child or family therapist who has experience with life-threatening illnesses.

An expert in the field can help you evaluate different ways to help your children, giving you another pair of eyes to analyze and assess your situation. It can't hurt to have someone to bounce ideas off of or to ask about parenting techniques. And having an objective outsider gives your kids a forum, a special coach whom they can confide in in a nonjudgmental, safe environment.

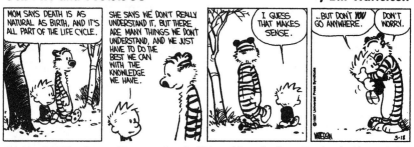

The most important reason I can give you to go to counseling is that it will affect the rest of your child's life. Many adults have said to me, "I wish we had gone to counseling when I went through this as a child." Many said that the way the cancer was handled in their homes led to an inability to have healthy adult relationships, psychosomatic illnesses, problems at work, or negative attitudes toward authority figures.

I will never forget Julianne, who came to a support group because her husband had cancer. Seven months into the group, she broke down crying. All the feelings that she hadn't dealt with about her mother's death came flooding back. Not until her husband was ill did she even realize how angry and bitter she still was, how many areas of her life it had affected. At forty-nine, she wrote each of her parents (who had died only a few years before) an imaginary letter, forgiving them for the way they treated her.

"These problems," Julianne said, "never had to happen. It didn't have to be this way. All these years of pain could have been prevented. I would always have missed her, but I would never have been so angry at my parents if they had just talked to me or taken us to counseling. This is not going to happen with my sons."

Her support group met six years ago. Today Julianne's sons do not exhibit the anger and pain their mother experienced.

When illness strikes, you deal with your pain and your old losses and fears. It is hard to handle those issues on top of your kids' problems. Outside help can become crucial.

Dr. Donna Copeland strongly advises people to find a counselor by obtaining a referral from another professional. "If a family sees someone who is not qualified, they may end up with more problems. I have heard of counselors attributing issues to an illness that are not related. They were preexisting family issues. The disease may have played into it, but it wasn't the main source of the problem. I have heard of therapists discussing topics that the family wasn't ready to talk about or didn't need to discuss."

When you call an organization for a referral, say, "I'm looking for a social worker, psychologist, or psychiatrist who has at least five years of experience working with children and serious illnesses. Can you give me the names of three people whom you have referred to before? Can you tell me a little bit about each one?" Call:

- A nearby graduate school of psychology, psychiatry, or social work will have a director of training, a professional who supervises students personally and has firsthand knowledge of their skills. They also are acquainted with professionals with whom they have placed their students for training. They aren't going to place a student with anyone who isn't well respected in the profession.
- Each of the agencies and hospitals listed in the Resources section of this book will have a director of social work, psychiatry, or psychology. You could also ask if they know a child life specialist. Dr. Copeland explains, "These specialists provide play therapy and support. They are certified, and many do have master's degrees in social work and counseling."

8. Involve school personnel.

Teachers and school counselors can be great allies for you and your kids. Many are qualified to provide counseling, support, and guidance for children. Make sure confidentiality is maintained between your child and school personnel.

Work with the counselor and teachers to educate your child's classmates. Ask the school to bring in a counselor who specializes in speaking to schools about coping with cancer.

9. Solicit help from relatives, friends, and Sunday school teachers.

These people can provide immeasurable comfort. Keep them updated on all medical progress. Be clear about what they can say to your children. Make sure they aren't being dishonest with them.

Ask them to be open, direct, and caring while maintaining hope. Explain how you are approaching the illness. If Daddy explains to the child that Mommy is getting worse, and then Grandma says, "But your Mommy will be just fine in a few weeks," the child will get confused. Whom is he supposed to trust?

Share this book with school counselors, baby-sitters, relatives, and others to whom your children may turn for help.

Practical Problems

10. Hold family meetings.

Dr. Mitch Golant recommends using family meetings to work out practical problems together. During these meetings family members can discuss what is reasonable and unreasonable to expect from one another. "The more parents are able to communicate," he says, "the more the children will communicate, and that is where solutions are created."

He recommends organizing meetings around one specific topic. The topic doesn't necessarily have to be resolved in one meeting. Meetings should last about twenty minutes. A short meeting is especially important for younger kids. "You can vary the length depending upon the ages," he says. "Regardless of the length, meetings shouldn't be interrupted."

During the meeting, Dr. Golant suggests the parents give each person in the family an opportunity to say their piece without being judged or criticized. "It's important for each person to have a say and be given consideration," he emphasizes. This nonjudgmental approach doesn't mean all the family members will agree or go along with every suggestion, but it does require them to listen to each other's point of view and to consider what they have to say. Suppose you say you want to plan a time each week when the family spends uninterrupted time engaging in a fun activity. You need to negotiate a schedule with your children. If your thirteen-year-old suggests Sunday mornings but no one else is available then, you can work together to find a more suitable time.

Let's say both parents have to go to another state for five days to get a second opinion. If the ten-year-old wants to stay at a friend's home and you know this particular friend's parents are never home, ask him to come up with another place he might stay.

Toward the end of the meeting, Dr. Golant recommends that you "move into problem-solving. Brainstorm solutions. If the problems aren't resolved, plan to meet again and follow up in a couple of nights. These meetings can become a regular family ritual or routine."

11. Delegate chores and find household help for larger projects whenever possible.

Children ought not to become parents and be put in charge of running a house. Yet they do have to do chores and participate in the household. They want you to need them, and they want to help. Still, it's one thing to ask your seven-year-old to help clean the dishes after dinner, and quite another to ask him to scrub the floors.

When Gary's wife had cancer, he asked her to make a list of projects the family could help her with. Then he held a family meeting and asked the children to select items they wanted to do for chores. He posted the list of chores on the refrigerator each week. He also hired a maid to come in once a week and a home health aide three times a week.

Call your volunteer center or United Way, and ask if they know of an agency whose volunteers will help with housekeeping. Some nursing agencies have reduced rates to help with bathing and taking care of patients' physical needs. Church members, neighbors, friends, and family members are also excellent resources.

12. Establish bedtime rituals.

If you already have bedtime rituals, great. If not, now is a good time to start. There are various possibilities: Read together at bedtime or talk about what your child has written in his journal or ask him to share his feelings about what happened that day. Even if a child is reluctant to share his feelings and all you do is read together, he may start to open up after you establish the ritual.

A woman whose thirty-two-year-old husband had cancer shared this story: "My girls wouldn't talk about their emotions. I knew they were trying to be brave, but no matter how much I encouraged them to open up, I failed. They kept journals, but they didn't discuss them with me.

"We had this ritual of reading together every night. I chose stories that I hoped would encourage them to talk about their feelings. That didn't work either. Then one evening as I was switching off the lights, one of them said, 'I was writing in my journal today. Would you like to see it?' We read a passage together, and from then on she was comfortable sharing her feelings." Rituals provide safe times for children to bring up their concerns.

13. Develop new ways to celebrate special occasions.

Writing letters to your children is a way you can express your love, your beliefs, and your dreams for them, without placing on them the burden of responding.

One mother used to put letters in her kids' Christmas stockings. Alongside the candy canes and treats was the treat they eventually treasured most of all. The contents of the letters varied—from hopes for the next year, to praise for something they did the year before, to sharing a childhood memory of her own.

When you are away and cannot attend an event, leave your child a letter. Imagine your lonely son as he is about to embark on the football game of his career. Before game time, he opens this letter of love and encouragement from you. How do you think he will feel? Or maybe he's been worried about a weekly test. When he comes home from studying, he finds your note beside his bed.

Special events can also be celebrated by taking children out in honor of their accomplishments. This provides time together and acknowledges their achievements.

Keep a scrapbook of all special events, holidays, and accomplishments. If a child's grades were good, put the report card in this book. If she wrote a wonderful essay, place one in the book. Frame the original and hang it on the wall.

Teach your children how to use the video camera, and encourage them to tape the events you are celebrating. Take still pictures of them with something that represents the event. Better yet, if you have more than one child, encourage them to take pictures of each other. Then show them how to set up their own photo album or help create a family photo album.

Ask your kids how they want to celebrate events. (Chapter 13 will give you more ideas for celebrations.)

14. Help the patient make a video for the children.

In the movie *My Life*, Michael Keaton (who is dying) makes a videotape while his wife is pregnant. In it he teaches his not-yet-born son how to shave, dance, greet someone at the door, shake hands at business meetings, and approach women.

People who have made videos for their kids say it is a way of passing themselves on to their children, while reliving their own lives. It can be a chronicle of one's life, a conversation about spiritual beliefs, or anything the patient wants the child to have. It doesn't matter what the prognosis is—the video will be treasured by the child for years.

15. Maintain discipline.

"Discipline is not a bad word if it's done in a loving way," says Dr. Copeland. Discipline is a form of love. If you stop disciplining a child, what message are you sending? If you don't maintain rules, your kids may think the cancer is worse than they thought because you don't care or have time enough to discipline them. For their own sake, keep setting clear limits and boundaries on their behavior.

Don't begin to accept bad behavior from them when a parent is ill. If they act poorly, say, "I love you, but you can't keep coming in late. You're grounded for the next two weeks." Or: "I love you, but I don't like it when you hurt other people in this house [or whatever the behavior is]."

Post the family rules in written form in a visible place, where other family members and baby-sitters can see them. Everyone has to be consistent about following your rules.

Helping Children Cope When the Patient Is Away from Home

16. Bring them to visit if they will benefit.

No single rule works for everyone about bringing children to a hospital, hospice, or any other patient facility. Each family has to weigh the benefits and consequences of a visit.

You have to respect the patient's wishes as well as the child's. The patient may think, "I don't want to be remembered this way," or "I look awful, and I don't want [the child] to see me."

If the patient objects to a child's visit, help him clarify his concerns. Say, "Let's talk about this. Is there a specific reason you don't want them to come? Are you afraid of how the children will react, or how they'll remember you, or how their visit will affect you?"

Verbalizing his feelings will help identify the patient's issues. After talking to you, he may change his mind. Conversely, he may be even more adamantly opposed to seeing the child. If, at the end of your discussion, he isn't sure how he feels, then ask him if he would like to

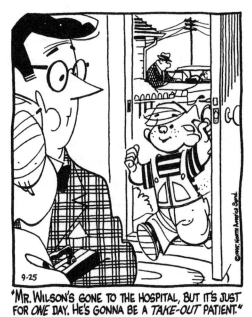

"MR. WILSON'S GONE TO THE HOSPITAL, BUT IT'S JUST FOR *ONE* DAY. HE'S GONNA BE A *TAKE-OUT* PATIENT."

Dennis The Menace® used by permission of Hank Ketcham and © by North America Syndicate.

speak to a professional who has experience helping families in this situation. If the situation is especially complicated, I'd encourage you to find out if the hospital has a child psychologist or medical ethicist on staff. These professionals have special training in addressing complicated issues such as bringing children to the hospital.

An outside counseling agency may also be of assistance. We were able to act as liaisons between families and hospitals. When a family was struggling with this or a similarly difficult decision, we'd call the hospital and schedule a meeting with staff members. And if the family didn't want to talk to the hospital staff, or if they already had and still hadn't reached a decision, we could consult with other specialists in the hospital on their behalf. (See the Resources section for names of agencies and therapists who may be able to provide similar services at no charge.)

When making your decision, weigh whether a visit will help or hurt the child. Never force a child to visit someone in a hospital. If the situation is at all questionable, then talk it over with a professional. If the children themselves don't want to go, help them verbalize their feelings. Perhaps they want to remember the patient as he was, or they may feel uncomfortable in a hospital because of a previous experience.

Dr. Judy Headley, the nursing professor whom we met in Chapter 4, observes that very young children think in concrete terms. It may be more important for them to visit a parent in the hospital because "if they can't see the parent, then they think the parent is gone. They need visual proof that the parent is alive."

If you decide against bringing the children to visit, you can still videotape the patient talking to them on camera. You can also bring home pictures or letters from the patient. If the patient is capable, arrange for regular telephone calls between the patient and the children.

If the patient is comfortable, peaceful, and not in distress or terrible pain, then, in general, children can benefit from a hospital visit. Visits can bring children and patients closer. Thousands of these visits, even those that were initially difficult to arrange, have become touching, beneficial, intimate experiences for both patients and their children.

I know of children who came to say good-bye to parents who were in comas or heavily sedated, and of children who visited patients in hospices. I have visited homes in which children lived alongside dying parents. In many cultures this is part of life. If you approach it as such, your children will be better able to cope with it. To make contact with a comatose patient easier and more meaningful, Dr. Headley recommends that you tell visiting children, "It's okay to talk to the patient. She'll hear you." She also says you should encourage the children to touch the patient's arms or hands.

17. Be prepared for a reaction during a visit.

Dr. Donna Copeland remembers when a family asked her whether they ought to bring their seven-year-old son to see his mother in intensive care. "She was hooked up to machines, and she had changed a lot. The family members were worried. Together we decided it would benefit the child to come to the hospital. Then we asked the boy if he wanted to visit. He did. When they brought him up, he walked into the room and whispered, 'Ahhhh . . . she looks so beautiful.'

"He didn't see the machines as we would because he didn't understand the meaning of them. He only knew he was being deprived of somebody important. He paid attention only to what he cared about, Mommy."

My two-year-old nephew, James, came to the hospital three days after my mother had her lung removed. She had not lost her trademark rosy-colored cheeks, and on that day she was quite animated. Medication had eased the pain.

I can't tell you she made absolute sense, and to this day we joke about the things she said, but to a child, all he saw was his grandma. Even now my mother brightens when she remembers James's reactions. "Children don't see things as we do," she says, "and he was fascinated with the equipment, rather than threatened by it or frightened. I still remember him absorbed with how the bed worked."

Children can also introduce humor into a difficult situation. James yanked down the small TV in my mother's room and proceeded to delight everyone there with his running commentary on the basketball playoffs, proudly pointing out Michael Jordan. Children have a way of interjecting joy, laughter, and a sense of innocence and awe into very stressful situations.

I don't want to leave you with the impression that hospital visits are always easy. My mother looked no different from the way she had looked the last time James had seen her. In Dr. Copeland's story the patient seemed peaceful to her child. Nevertheless, when a patient looks very different or is hooked up to machines or is uncomfortable, it can be very scary to some children. It's important to tell your children ahead of time that it might be scary so there aren't any big shocks. You can say, "It might be scary when you are in there, but remember Mommy loves you, and the doctors are taking good care of her and keeping her comfortable." Dr. Brendan O'Rourke says such messages empower a child to accept his feelings. "Once a child is in the room, give him something to do. 'You can stand by Mommy or let her hear your voice.'"

The adults in the room, be they the patients or relatives, may be extremely tense during a visit. Children can pick up that tension and become uncomfortable or scared. It's important that you try to remain calm.

Last year I brought my six-month-old daughter to see my grandmother, who had been ill for two years. Laughing, my grandmother devoured every moment watching the antics of her great-granddaughter. She died two months later. My daughter had had ear infections when my grandmother was in hospice, but if she hadn't, I wouldn't have hesitated to bring her to visit. As Lars Egede-Nissen, executive director of the hospice at the Texas Medical Center, explains, "In-patient hospices are usually set up like comfortable homes, and children feel comfortable visiting. If you're not sure about the facility, you can always tour it before you bring a child."

Another service that hospice provides is counseling. Most hospice teams who provide either in-patient or homebound services consist of social workers and chaplains. You may want to talk to these professionals about how to support your children and how to make the most of the time they spend with the patient. As Egede-Nissen explains, "We are able to ease a family's emotional and spiritual pain and guide them through the patient's final journey."

18. Plan for the visit.

Once you have decided to go to the hospital, engage your children in planning the visit. Help them choose a gift for the patient, or draw a picture, or write a poem for the hospital room.

Ask if the hospital has a child life specialist, a child psychologist, or a social worker who can help your children prepare. These professionals will often walk a child through procedures, explaining what transpires at the hospital.

You can buy a medical kit and dress dolls up as hospital personnel.

Using dolls, children can act out and discuss their feelings about going to the hospital. Playing doctor helps them understand the situation. For younger children, describe what the environment looks like. "Mommy's in the hospital. She looks very different." While you are explaining, show them photographs of the outside of the hospital, the patient, the room, and the bed. You can take these pictures yourself or use a hospital brochure. The more accurate the picture, the more prepared the child will be.

There are many ways a patient can make children feel comfortable when they visit. Help the patient decide on a gift to give them. It doesn't have to be elaborate, but it will mean a lot. Or ask the patient if he would like to place something in his room that shows he thinks about the children—their cards, drawings, awards, or pictures. Dr. Judy Headley recalls a parent who displayed her ten-year-old's picture next to the hospital bed. "When the daughter saw the picture, she realized her mom had not forgotten her."

After the visit, do something quiet and easy. Go for a ride, for ice cream, to a park, or whatever your children suggest. Later, ask the younger kids to draw a picture of what it was like to visit the hospital. You could ask the teenagers to discuss it or to write a letter to a friend about the visit.

A visit that is well prepared for can have numerous beneficial results. Most important, it can allay children's fears. The husband of one patient explains, "After visiting his mother, my nine-year-old was less frightened about where Mommy was. Now when I visit my wife in the hospital, he knows where I am. He isn't wondering anymore. He told me the hospital wasn't as bad as he thought it was going to be, and Mommy looked better than he imagined."

A visit can bring a patient and a child closer. It can help the child understand what is happening to someone he loves. It can make him feel as though he did something concrete to help. After visiting his father, a nine-year-old turned to his mother and said, "Aren't you glad we went? Daddy really needed us to cheer him up." The mother told me, "It was the first time I had heard either of them laugh in weeks."

19. If the patient's treatment is far away, leave children at home whenever possible, except for short visits.

It's important to maintain normalcy as much as possible. Uprooting children may require them to make too much of an adjustment and it robs them of their friends and support systems. Plopping them down in a hotel room or with someone they hardly know in a strange city can be especially hard.

Children do best when they stay home and maintain a sense of connection with the absent parent in other ways. Let them take turns making phone calls. They can make audio- and videotapes of their activities. I will never forget a video that one family from out of state showed us. Their four kids had gone to great lengths to cheer their parents up. The video showed one child holding up his report card and beaming into the camera, proud of his good news. Two of the children performed a skit. The eldest child gave a commentary on his latest basketball game, acting as if he were a radio announcer. With a brush in one hand and his other hand over his ear, he described the game play-by-play.

Encourage your children to write letters. A friend can help them pick out humorous cards. Children can also take pictures of their activities and send them with notes attached.

If the patient is going to be away for a month or so, you could bring the children to visit for a few days. Decide when would be the best time. If the patient has three months of out-of-state chemotherapy, a weekend every three or four weeks might be optimal. If the children are under ten years old, you could bring them to visit during school holidays. But children of any age who have a well-established network of friends may need to spend those holidays with their friends. If the patient does not want to see the children that often or isn't up to seeing them, then you could also return home for a few days at regular intervals. This is something you might want to discuss with the patient before she leaves. It's a good topic for a family meeting.

Help your children prepare a welcome-home party for when the parent returns. If you cannot be there, ask a relative or close friend to help them with it. Kids can bake cookies, make welcome-home banners, and help decorate the house.

The Most Important Keys

20. Never forget they are children—don't let them grow up too fast.

Your children are not there to take care of you. You are there to take care of them. Harvey Aronson, a social worker on staff at Cancer Counseling who has more than fifteen years' experience working with kids affected by cancer, warns parents, "Don't let your kids become *parentfied.*" Your kids can help out and take on responsibilities, but do not force them to become parents too soon. Let them be kids in every way possible.

"Be careful not to let one child become the caregiver of other children," Aronson warns. "Certain amounts of responsibilities are reasonable, but if you let a child become a parent, it may show up later as rebellious behavior or a diminished capacity for fun and joy."

21. Keep laughing, and make time for fun.

Time spent laughing with your children is crucial to their well-being and yours. Watch funny movies together. Tell funny stories, and point out the humor in your day-to-day activities. Make time to go to a matinee, a child's sports event, the zoo, a museum, a city activity, or a play. Go to the video store and let your children pick out movies. Get an ice cream, or take a walk together.

This disease will affect your children—there is no way to prevent it. Dealing with a catastrophic illness is never simple. There will be times when you lose your temper or they will lose theirs. There will be times when you cannot help them. As long as you do your best to be open, honest, and loving, they will grow in positive ways from this experience. Just remember, they want to be included, to help, to participate. They are traveling on this path with you.

Chapter 11

Finding the Best Doctors: What You Can Do Before the First Appointment

In 1982 Dr. Gerry Hogan came storming out of his office shaking his head. A worried family had just left, shuffling by me.

"See. See. This is why you need to set up that cancer agency," Dr. Hogan said to me, "for families like that one." He knew families like this all too well. For thirty-three years he had encountered numerous family members who did not participate in their loved one's care, who arrived only when the patient was dying or had to be placed in a nursing home or hospice.

It was out of character for Dr. Hogan to get frustrated. He was one of the most caring doctors I knew. He rubbed his head. "During three years of treatment, I never saw the family once. I never got a call, a letter—anything."

"Did they visit the patient?" I asked.

"I'm not sure. The patient was always very guarded about her relatives. She seemed pretty upset whenever I mentioned them.

"It doesn't matter," he continued. "They're here now. She's dying, and they're mad. They want an explanation, an answer, a miracle. They barged into my office this morning screaming at me. Besides admitting her to a hospice, we now have to address the dissension between family members."

Dr. Hogan was not begrudging this family their concerns—he was only frustrated because they had chosen to voice them at such a late date. "Had they been active and informed," he said, "they would have spared us all the confusion and frustration we are now facing."

Like so many physicians, Dr. Hogan has been on various sides of the cancer battle. He has been a professor, conducted research, and led community cancer organizations. He has watched his mother, sister, friends, and colleagues fight the disease. We forget that doctors are people too, dealing with this illness not only as physicians but as sons, brothers, and sometimes patients themselves.

"If I can ease the burdens of my patients, extend their lives, or at least ensure that they get the best care available, then I have done my job well," said Dr. Hogan.

As you and your loved ones enter the hallways of any hospital, you will meet physicians like Dr. Hogan. Of course, not all doctors are good communicators. This chapter will teach you how to find a doctor whom the patient can communicate with and trust. You'll learn how to maximize the time she spends with the physician in order to build a mutually beneficial relationship. As in most relationships, there will be times when she and the doctor do not get along. You cannot change the fact that sometimes any doctor will be rushed or preoccupied. But you can help the patient understand and appreciate how doctors work best. Families who are considerate of doctors will have a better chance of getting along with them than will those who storm in demanding answers. If you're the patient, this chapter will enable you to find the best doctors and prepare for your appointments. You may also want to share this chapter with whomever you bring to your appointments with you.

I have worked with hundreds of doctors, and for this chapter I interviewed more than sixty physicians at various cancer centers and hospitals, asking them how people can enhance the doctor-family relationship. I asked them what they appreciated and what drove them crazy. Their candid answers will give you and your loved ones some insights into how your doctor may be feeling.

When I asked, "What do families do that drive you crazy?" the most common answers I got, in no particular order, were:

> "Families that do not accompany the patient on regular visits, appearing only when there is a major problem."
>
> "Patients and family members who don't participate in the care we are trying to provide. They do not read the brochures or pamphlets I give them."
>
> "Patients and family members who compare themselves to neighbors or people they meet in my waiting room. Each patient is an individual, different from any other person who has cancer."
>
> "Patients and family members who see doctors and nurses as adversaries."
>
> "Patients who don't trust us after we've agreed to work together. I encourage families to get a second opinion before treatment starts. But once treatment starts, we're in this together, and there has to be a level of trust. If they run off every other week questioning my decisions, it's going to be difficult to work together."
>
> "Families who try to push patients into treatment they don't want."
>
> "Families who wait until the patient isn't around to ask me questions."
>
> "Families who are rude to my staff."

The behaviors doctors said they appreciated were:

> "Assertive patients and family members who come pre-pared with written questions, tape recorders, notes, and brief outlines of their complaints."
>
> "Patients who respect my time. I'm more than happy to schedule longer visits if they let my office know in advance. Tell my secretary, 'I'll be needing an extra half hour to go over some concerns I have.' 'I'll be needing an extra forty-five minutes because my husband is coming to this visit, and I want the doctor to discuss my care in depth.' "
>
> "Patients who are honest about their medical condition."
>
> "Families who let me know when they have a problem with something I've said or with the way I communicate."
>
> "Family members who respect patients' wishes."
>
> "Someone who says thank you."
>
> "Patients who bring an easy-to-read outline of their history on the first visit, including dates of major operations and illnesses. Medical records, X rays, and reports from previous tests are also helpful."
>
> "A family who wants to work as a team with me."
>
> "Families who share resources, books, and ideas that I can investigate and pass on to my other patients."
>
> "Families who tell me they have a handwritten list of questions at the beginning of the visit."

The best way to find out how your doctor wants to approach your relationship is to ask him directly. You may think how he feels doesn't matter, but as in any relationship, understanding how he feels allows you to make compromises to get along with him. If your spouse hates it when you leave your shoes and clothes strewn around the house, then once in a while you just might pick up those shoes. It may be a compromise, but you will save *yourself* the frustration of listening to his complaints.

Joining the Alliance

Many families today are learning that they can secure the best medical care by becoming their own advocates. They are assertive about their needs and open to possibilities, and they seek out new opportunities.

Regardless of what kind of relationship you have with your medical professional, you can always improve it. The person who benefits most of all will be the patient. But you both will reap the rewards of a positive working relationship with those caring for him.

The best way to achieve a good relationship is to start by talking with the patient about how you both want to deal with doctors. You ought to agree on how your family is going to handle appointments, phone calls, and information.

If you are a loved one, your way of handling difficult situations may differ from the patient's. You have to respect the patient's style. He should be the one to take the lead with the health care team. He has the primary responsibility for his care. He has to be in charge of the direction and tone it takes.

This chapter and the next one will show patients and loved ones how to strengthen relationships with doctors and other medical professionals. In addition, they will teach you how to find resources. If the patient does not agree with your suggestions, then respect her wishes. She has to be in charge of her care to every degree possible. Your job is to assist her, not to direct her.

First Things First: Starting Out

Discuss your coping styles.

"Discuss what the disease means to both of you," suggests Dr. Stratton Hill, a world-renowned expert on pain management. He advises family members and patients to write down their concepts of the disease and review them with their doctors.

In thirty-two years of practice, he has found that "patients and their loved ones can have completely different ideas about treatments and outcomes than their physicians. Talking about how families view the disease can help us clear up misunderstandings." An additional benefit of following this advice, advises Dr. Hill, "is it will also help families understand their feelings."

Before you go to the doctor, ask yourself the following questions to identify your way of coping:

- How much do I need to know?
- How much do I want to know?
- Do I have any preconceived fears?
- Are you afraid of certain treatments because of a previous experience? (If you inform your doctor of any fears at the outset, he will be aware of how this treatment will affect you. The doctor must take these fears seriously.)
- What if the treatment does not work?
- What will the patient be like after treatment?
- How will it affect our relationship?
- How do I expect the patient to respond to treatment?

Merry Templeton, a volunteer from the American Cancer Society, shares a story about a couple who didn't discuss this last question about expectations for treatment: "The husband was on a business trip and had a long drive home. During the ride he thought about his wife's cancer. The doctors were optimistic that they could achieve a cure. Unfortunately, he did not believe them. By the time he got home," Merry said, "he thought she was going to die." As a result, he withdrew from his wife. And she felt as if he didn't care about her. This couple ended up pulling away from each other because he didn't tell her what his expectations were. Had he explained them, the problem could have been resolved.

Ask the patient if she wants patient education materials.

The more families and patients understand, the more in control they will feel and the more qualified they will be to make decisions.

Greg Fredo, chair of the Information Resources Task Force of the National Cancer Institute's Cancer Information Service, advises, "Part of your role as caregiver can be to assist the patient in gathering information."

Social worker Allison Stovall, from M. D. Anderson Cancer Center, adds: "Before you run around getting information, ask the patient what he wants. Say, 'I want to get materials about the disease. I am going to the library—do you want me to get copies for you?' Or: 'I don't mind getting extra brochures. You may not want to read them now, but they will be here in case you are interested later.'"

Include the patient in treatment decisions.

Dr. Garrett Walsh, an M. D. Anderson Cancer Center surgeon, explains: "Too many families come to me with the intention of excluding the patient from the planning of treatment. I realize they are doing what they think is best, but I won't treat patients without their full understanding of what I am doing. I also find when patients participate in their care, they do better medically and recover more quickly."

Dr. Eugene Carlton, ninetieth president of the American Urological Association, agrees: "There shouldn't be anything a family member asks the doctor that he can't tell the patient. It's to the family's benefit if they all listen to me at the same time. It helps them to get 'on the same page,' even though they are in different places emotionally.

"When there isn't communication, there is tension, a conspiracy of silence. For example, when a wife follows me into the hall and says, 'I have some questions, but I don't want to ask them in front of my husband,' I walk her back in and discuss her concerns in front of him. If we work together, they have a better chance of solving their problems."

Before you go to a doctor, decide what you will do if the patient is saturated with information but you still have more questions. Ask the patient if he will allow you and the doctor to meet alone. During the meeting, no new disclosures should be made. You should only review what the physician has discussed before. If you want to bring up something new, ask yourself how you would feel if a family member knew more about your disease than you did. I've had family members tape these meetings and hand them over to patients.

During a speech at Barry College in Florida in 1980, Dr. Elisabeth Kübler-Ross explained how parents try to protect children who have cancer. They withhold information to "help" their kids. When Dr. Kübler-Ross talked to the children herself or had them draw pictures about their illness, she realized that they clearly understood what was wrong with them. They did not need to be protected. Most adult patients feel the same way. They know what is wrong, and they may even handle the news better than their loved ones.

Assign a point person.

"Families should assign one member to talk to their doctor—a point person," Dr. Hill explains. "That person can keep the others updated." Dr. Raphael Pollock, who serves on the Executive Council of the Society for Surgical Oncology and on the Commission on Cancer of the American College of Surgeons, adds, "This arrangement saves doctors hours of time that we can better use to treat patients. It also identifies who the patient wants me to talk to in the case of an emergency." Assigning one person to disseminate information will reduce misunderstanding among family members and lessen the chances that they will hear contradictory medical information.

Dr. Gabriel Hortobagyi, president of the Ninth Conference on Breast Diseases, adds, "The point person should be carefully chosen on the basis of being assertive, relating well to people, being a problem solver, and having the ability to communicate clearly."

The point person should be the person the patient feels most comfortable with—not necessarily the obvious person. If a couple is estranged, the spouse may want a sibling, friend, or parent as the point person. Allison Stovall adds, "Ideally, the point person should be the one who has the durable power of attorney." The durable power of attorney for health care, or the health proxy, enables a patient to authorize an individual to make health care decisions for her in the event she herself cannot make informed medical choices.

Tell the doctor who the patient's point person is. When family members call, doctors can refer them to this person.

Get information.

Doctors and Their Staffs

One of the first places to turn when you are searching for information should be the patient's doctor, nurses, or physician's assistants. They have the patient's records, and they know the details of his history. They have the facts regarding the prognosis and treatment.

Dr. Raphael Pollock recommends how best to use this resource: "If a patient or family isn't comfortable asking me questions, then I encourage them to discuss their concerns with my physician's assistant or nurse. They can answer questions and show the family where to get brochures or articles."

Before you start your research, ask the doctor or his staff for help. Say: "We'd like to do a search of the literature. Can you tell us details about our case that we'll need to know? Can you suggest publications to review? Are there any specific articles or books you'd recommend?"

The National Cancer Institute's Cancer Information Service (800-4-CANCER)

Ask the CIS to send you their free pamphlets about the medical and psychological aspects of cancer. Inquire about PDQ (Physician Data Query), a free database that contains state-of-the-art cancer treatment information; lists more than three thousand organizations that provide cancer care programs; identifies researchers performing clinical trials; and provides facts on some investigational and newly approved anticancer drugs and ways to treat cancer-related symptoms such as nausea. Every month, PDQ's editorial boards review this database. PDQ does not recommend one treatment over another but describes treatment options. Doctors, patients, and loved ones use PDQ to learn about the best treatments currently available.

CIS's professionals will answer your questions and discuss your concerns about the disease, but they cannot give you medical advice. They also have one of the best referral services to other community and health-related resources.

Hospital Libraries

Most major hospitals have a comprehensive library, with tapes, brochures, books, and articles. In addition, some keep current lists of community resources. Call your hospital's social work department or your doctor's secretary, and ask if the hospital has such a library. Or use a hospital library affiliated with a teaching school or medical center.

Medical School Libraries

You probably will not be able to check out books from a medical school library, but you can usually get assistance in locating and reviewing materials. However, if you ask the librarian to help you research lung cancer, you could become overwhelmed by the scope and technical level of information. Much of the information may not have anything to do with your loved one's situation. Before you go to the library, talk to your doctor or the professionals at CIS. They can save you time and teach you how to research relevant materials.

Your local American Cancer Society, (800) ACS-2345

The American Cancer Society (ACS), a voluntary nationwide service, has fifty-seven divisions and 3,400 local units providing education and referrals. They offer an extensive set of free brochures, articles, and pamphlets. Some of their brochures include *Caring for the Patient with Cancer at Home, Look Good, Feel Better: Caring for Yourself Inside and Out,* and *I Can Cope,* which lists a series of classes they conduct. In Texas they have a superb pamphlet called *Keys to Services.* It lists everything from housing to counseling resources. Ask your local ACS unit if they have a similar brochure on community resources.

Health Information Online

"Was there a reason you left out clinical trial X when you posted new studies?" I asked the authors of one well-respected site.

They looked at the study I was holding and said, "Oh, that one is much better than what we have on the site, but it's not as readily available. We didn't list it because we didn't want to give people false hope."

The study I was referring to (clinical trial X) was not posted on four other national sites. Yet the two leading cancer centers were among the places this trial had openings.

The Internet provides information, not treatment. Even the best sites may not carry all the information or treatments available. Therefore, do not substitute navigating the Net for talking with your doctor or other specialists. When you find reputable, encouraging information, bring it to your doctor to review. Print a summary of the information and note where you obtained it. Your doctor knows your history. He may be able to help you assess if a study you are interested in is beneficial. Some doctors will assist you in getting admitted to a study you find. A good starting point for your research are the resources at the back of this book, along with medical school sites and media web sites that post breaking news.

When doing research on the Internet regarding resources, alternative medicine, or new treatments, keep these questions in mind:

- Have you checked the NEWS section and the archives? A new FDA-approved treatment appeared in the news section of one site but did not show up on other areas of the site for nine months. Clinical trial X above did not appear on any site except the *Wall Street Journal*'s site for six months.
- Can you find a staff page that gives the names, affiliations, and degrees of the professionals overseeing the site? Will they for-

ward you literature about the site? If they won't, or don't have email, that's a reason to be suspicious.

- Is the site asking too many personal questions? Do not give out your social security number or mother's maiden name. Leave a site that asks for that kind of information.
- Do they have self interests in the stories, remedies, or treatments they promote?
- Do they encourage you to search other sites or claim they have the only answer? Good sites have links to other sites because they want to provide as much information as possible.
- Have they received any awards? What are the criteria of the award? Do you recognize the sponsor?
- How often is the site updated? Is the article you are reading recent? Can you contact the author? If so, does he return your email?
- Do they offer personalized medical advice? Unless they have all of your information and have examined you, it's difficult to give a full assessment. Doctors on the web may give you some good ideas, but always check with your doctor.
- Are the sites—especially those that aren't well known—policed by the Health On the Net Foundation? They've developed the HONcode of conduct to help standardize the reliability of medical and health information available on the Internet. The HONcode is not an award system, nor does it intend to rate the quality of the information provided by the web site. It only defines a set of rules to hold web site developers to basic ethical standards in the presentation of information and to help make sure the readers always know the source and purpose of the data they are reading.
- Is the information backed by an authoritative source or credible sources you can recognize?
- Are claims backed up with scientific studies that have appeared in peer-reviewed journals? If so, you may want to find the original article on Medline.com and print the abstracts and studies. Show your doctor the abstract, which should briefly answer the

basic questions posed by a study. Have the entire study with you in case he wants to look at it in detail.

Mention the sites you visit to your doctor and see if she knows about them and ask her for sites she recommends. Ask the nurse, people on the staff, and members of your support group for their favorite sites.

If you are trying to find a doctor, beware of the online "best doctor" lists. Always use the method in this book as a research tool for finding a doctor before spending money on someone just because they appear on a web site. In a survey of four of these sites, three of the most respected doctors in cancer care and a leading cardiologist, Dr. Denton Cooley, weren't listed. A doctor who provided the worst care I've observed in years was.

There are excellent doctors listed on these sites. The sites are worthwhile resources if you do your own research after reviewing what they offer.

The Internet is a starting point. It offers the latest treatments; up-to-date news, in-depth information about therapies your doctors may prescribe, alternative treatments, and a wealth of resources, such as bulletin boards, chat sessions, and articles about all aspects of your disease. The Internet is an invaluable tool that can help you make informed, accurate medical decisions and offer psychological, practical, and social support when you use it with caution.

Community Agencies

Community organizations work closely with patients, family members, and their health care professionals. They often teach families how to identify issues, help them develop questions for their doctors, show them where to get literature, secure outside services, and work directly with health care providers. Many publish a free newsletter and numerous health-related materials.

The phone numbers and web sites of health care agencies are listed in the Resources section. When you call an agency, ask for information on any free programs or brochures they provide. Always check the date of a medical brochure to make sure the information is current.

Finding a Physician

Your loved one may ask you to check the credentials of his doctor. You can also help him research doctors for a second opinion. These sources can get you started:

MEDICAL SOCIETIES

Dr. Charles A. LeMaistre, 1986 president of the American Cancer Society and former president of the M. D. Anderson Cancer Center, suggests you "call your local medical society and ask about the physician's training and experience. Verify that she is in good standing in the medical community."

DEPARTMENT CHAIRPERSONS AND PROFESSORS

Contact heads of departments and professors at medical schools. When you reach the school or center, ask for the chairman or a professor of gynecology, urology, internal medicine, family practice, surgery, or psychiatry. These specialists interact with their colleagues across the country and are familiar with their reputations.

Ask the secretary if the chairperson or professor will comment on your list of prospective doctors. When I showed a list of doctors to a physician from California, he said, "I can look over the list and at least recommend a name I am familiar with, without commenting on others."

When my grandfather had cancer a few months ago, I called Dr. David Robinson, associate professor of surgery at the University of Miami Medical School, to ask about Dr. Jerome Spunberg, who practices in Palm Beach County. Although Dr. Spunberg lives more than an hour away and they practice in different areas of medicine, Dr. Robinson not only knew him, he said he would send his family to him. A recommendation like this can be very reassuring.

DOCTORS YOU RESPECT

Ask for referrals from a doctor you respect. When you reach her, ask whom she sent her own family members to. Another good question is, "Where would you go if you had this diagnosis?"

MEDICAL ORGANIZATIONS

Some medical organizations will tell you only if the name you give them is a member or a fellow of their organization. Others will also provide referrals to qualified practitioners. Specific resources include:

American College of Radiologists, (800) 227-5463, www.acr.org
American Board of Medical Specialists, (866) ASK-ABMS, www.abms.org
American College of Surgeons, (312) 202-5000, www.fucs.org

When you call, ask for the office of public information. Kim DiGangi, who works for the College of Surgeons, suggests that you call the referral service at the hospital where the doctor practices. Ask what societies the doctor belongs to. Then call the societies to find out if the doctor is a member or a fellow.

If a doctor is not a member of one of these organizations, she may be a member of a surgical subspecialty organization, such as the Society of Surgical Oncology or the American Association for Thoracic Surgery. DiGangi's office will provide you with phone numbers for these subspecialty organizations.

Board certification does assure a level of competence, but some good doctors who are older are not board certified. Certification has become important only since the 1970s. If your physician is not certified, evaluate where he practices, what his colleagues think of him, if he is respected in his local medical community, or if he is affiliated with a medical school or an NCI Comprehensive Cancer Center.

I went through the suggestions listed here when I was researching Dr. Spunberg. I discovered that he had references from peers, had trained at Harvard Medical School, had served on the Board of the

Susan G. Komen Breast Cancer Foundation, and had been president of the Palm Beach County division of the American Cancer Society.

What was most important about Dr. Spunberg, though, was that my grandfather respected, liked, and trusted him. Working with him contributed to the positive attitude my grandfather maintained during weeks of radiation treatments.

Preparing for the Visit

Get medical records ahead of time.

Dr. Gabriel Hortobagyi advises: "It is very helpful to your physician if he has an accurate, concise, up-to-date summary of the patient's care up until the visit. Some patients show up with several pounds of photocopies of charts. It might take hours to extract the important information and organize it in a useful way. Time spent on this activity is taken away from direct face-to-face contact time."

Have all tests, including slides, sent to the doctor ahead of your first visit. If the patient prefers to bring slides, reports, and X rays along personally, ask her to sign a release authorizing you to pick them up. Bring copies of any blood tests or written reports. Call the doctor's office and ask him what tests the patient should bring.

Set up a complete record.

Being prepared will reduce some of the stress associated with an initial visit. The better prepared you both are, the more in control you will feel. As a result, you will leave the doctor's office with more information and more knowledge. Being prepared empowers patients to make informed decisions.

Dr. Eugene Carlton suggests you "help your loved one make a list of topics you both want to discuss. When he gets to the doctor, he can always say, 'I'm not worried about these things, but my wife is.'"

It's helpful to set up a notebook to organize records and questions in one convenient place. Ask the patient if she would like you to buy an easy-to-carry loose-leaf notebook or get one herself. Let her set up the notebook herself. Here is the structure that my patients have found to be most effective. If she wants the notebook but does not want to organize it, ask her to highlight the topics that follow which she would like to include. Then you can type in or neatly write in the topics she has chosen.

Tab 1: What to Ask on the First Visit

Roger, the patient from Chapter 3 who told his wife his symptoms but not his doctor, like many other patients, is more comfortable handing the doctor a list of his symptoms or questions. This saves time because the doctor can quickly read over the list and then address them in an appropriate order. Alternatively, the patient could read the questions, unless she insists you ask them or she is not capable.

Families who use these techniques say they inject some objectivity into their visits. Placing structure on the situation eases tension. Once the patient feels comfortable, she can ask additional clarifying questions.

Here are some questions the patient may want to ask:

> "At what hospital, facility, or medical center do you per-
> form tests and admit patients?"
> "Who answers your calls when you are not on duty?"
> "How long have you been in practice?"
> "How many of these procedures do you do a year?"

Besides being a qualified doctor, Dr. Garrett Walsh, a thoracic surgeon at M. D. Anderson Cancer Center, operates on two to three hundred patients a year and has operated on thousands of people since he began his practice. I would rather have a doctor with his experience than a doctor who performs the *same* procedure only once or twice a year.

> "How long will it take to make a diagnosis?"
> "Will you review any studies about treatment that we
> find?"

"Will you recommend a doctor for a second opinion if
we want one?"
"Do you have any colleagues at major medical schools
or cancer centers who could tell us more about you?"
"Have you taught at a medical school?"
"Will you consult with colleagues in other institutions
about my case?"

There are excellent physicians throughout the country who have
trained at prestigious medical schools, been on staff at comprehensive
cancer centers, or taught at teaching hospitals. Some of the finest
doctors I know then left the major centers because they were state-
funded and did not permit them to have a private practice. Others
left to set up a practice in a rural area, to avoid a long commute. Still
other doctors just didn't want to be part of a large institution. Many
of these physicians still consult with colleagues at cancer centers and
prestigious medical centers.

Tab 2: What to Ask If the Doctor Requests Tests

Keep several copies of this list in the notebook.

"If [the patient] has already taken this test, can you
use the previous one?"
"Can you explain what the test is like?"
"How long does it take?"
"How accurate is it?"
"What are the risks? What are the benefits?"
"Is there a comparable test that takes less time or that
has fewer risks?"
"Is the test necessary? Is it being used as a baseline to
measure future results?"
"How does [the patient] prepare for the test?"
"How soon can [the patient] return to normal activi-

ties?" Tell the doctor what the patient's normal activities are. Is he lifting heavy materials or a child? Does he sit or drive for long periods of time?

"Will someone have to drive [the patient] home afterward?"

"When will someone call us with the results?"

"If the purpose of the test is to evaluate various treatment options, how long can we take to decide which one we will use?"

"What methods do you have to treat the side effects?"

"What are the normal results for this test?"

Tab 3: What to Ask When Treatment Is Recommended

"What are the side effects of the treatment?"

"Will it affect sleeping, concentration, strength, eating, eyesight, fertility, or sexual functioning?"

"Will it affect other areas of my life?"

"What tests will you do to determine if the treatment is working? How often?"

"How soon will you know if the treatment is working?"

"What are the best and worst possible results of this treatment?"

"How long will it take?"

"Is [the patient] eligible for a clinical trial instead of or in conjunction with the therapy?"

"Will this treatment make me ineligible for other treatments?"

"Will it extend [the patient's] life?"

"Do you have any pamphlets on the treatment or its side effects?"

"Do you know where I can find out more about the treatment?"

"Can we schedule the treatment without interfering

with our other plans [for an out-of-state wedding, a family function, or a long-awaited trip] or during mornings instead of afternoons?"

"If we travel, can you give us out-of-town contacts to administer treatment?"

"Can you give us contacts for emergencies?"

"What is the ten-year survival rate for this procedure?"

"What symptoms do we need to watch out for that would indicate we should return home for a medical follow-up?"

"How soon do we have to decide to do it?"

Tab 4: Symptoms

The patient should keep a list of symptoms. Date the top of each entry, and list each symptom when it occurs. Update the list as needed.

Symptoms include any physiological changes and any altered patterns of eating or sleeping. Include as well any changes in daily activities. If the symptom lasts several days, make a note of it: "February 4: Slept briefly in afternoons but not at night." "March 10: Trouble concentrating."

A scale will assign an objective measurement to symptoms that are often hard to describe. On a scale of one to ten, the patient should rate his level of pain. If the pain is not always located in one particular place, record where it is located. When he records his symptoms, he can write, "February 4: The pain was a 6 for most of the day." He can use letter abbreviations, such as P for *pain* and different letters for the locations: "L shoulder P, all day." "Back and neck P, 7 A.M.–3 P.M."

This record of symptoms will inform the doctor of the level and location of pain in the days and weeks before he sees the patient.

The more the patient communicates about his symptoms, the better equipped the doctor will be to provide treatment. Doctors know only as much as patients tell them.

Tab 5: Medications

Keep a list of all medications (including dosage) that the patient takes. Before the first visit, list all of them, including vitamins, herbal supplements, and over-the-counter drugs. When the doctor discontinues a prescription, cross it off the list. When she adds a new one, jot it down along with the date the patient started it. You might want to keep a copy of this list on your hand-held organizer.

Tab 6: Important Documents

Include the following documents in the notebook:

- A brief, up-to-date outline of the patient's medical history, including any allergies. List all illnesses and surgeries in chronological order.
- The names, addresses, phone numbers, and fax numbers of any outside health care providers, home health care services, counselors, rehabilitation centers, hospice personnel, or support groups.
- The names and phone numbers of auxiliary hospital services, social workers, nurses, volunteers, and chaplains.
- A copy of the durable power of attorney, the name of your Health Care Agent, and the living will. The living will states the patient's wishes for end of life care. (You can print out a living will for no charge at partnershipforcaring.org). The social work department at your hospital, your attorney, or the local bar association can make copies of these documents available to you. They may also assist you in filling them out.
- Insurance policy and names of insurance company representatives and hospital billing personnel.
- Names and phone numbers of departments you contact on a regular basis, including the number of the nurses' station if the patient is hospitalized.
- A copy of all legal documents. A second copy should go in your files, and the originals should be kept in a safe-deposit box. You may also want to send copies to your attorney, adult children, siblings, or parents.

Tab 7: Miscellaneous

This section is for questions that arise between visits. Date each entry.

The patient may want to keep this section in a small notepad, one that fits in a pocket in the notebook. She can keep this notepad by her bed or carry it with her, to write down questions as they arise. Insert the notepad into the notebook before doctors' visits.

This notebook will help your family keep medical information and records in one place. If there is a crisis, they will have immediate access to potentially life-saving information for emergency personnel. Take the notebook with you when you and the patient travel together.

Your loved one may have a home health care provider, hospice worker, or volunteer who stays with her when you are away. If this is the case, make sure this support person knows where the notebook is, in case of an emergency.

After you have organized your questions and completed your initial research, talk with the patient about how she wants to handle appointments. The next chapter gives you ways to make the most of doctors' visits. It also gives other resources. You may not avail yourselves of them immediately, but over the next weeks and months, they may become essential components of the patient's care.

Chapter 12

Building a Winning
Health Care Team

Some say luck is really a combination of intense preparation and the ability to spot opportunities. This chapter will teach you how to maximize the opportunities your family has to work with your health care team.

Before your loved one schedules his first appointments, he can learn how to prepare himself. You can help him do that. If he is well prepared, he will feel more in control and better able to focus on the most important issues.

Doctors and patients both possess unique insights into this disease. Planning ahead empowers a patient to work with her doctor in a way that facilitates the exchange of that information.

This chapter explains how to build a winning relationship with the doctor and how to enlist the support of other health care professionals. As with finding a doctor, you and your loved one have to determine how best to utilize these suggestions.

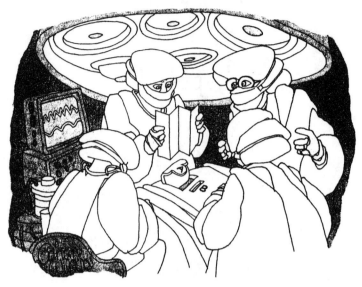

"O.K., now put Tab A into Slot B."

Drawing by Gahan Wilson; ©1991 The New Yorker Magazine, Inc.

Doctors' Appointments: How to Make Them More Productive

1. Decide ahead of time how to conduct appointments.

Ask the patient how she wants to cover issues with the doctor. You can offer to bring up any concerns she does not want to discuss. It is preferable, however, that she do as much of the talking as possible. It's also important that she feel comfortable with your behavior in the office. Some patients prefer that loved ones do not ask questions or interject comments. If this is how the patient feels and you do not agree, then you may not be the right person to attend appointments. If you do attend, respect the patient's wishes, and share any concerns you have with her in private. Ways to discuss these subjects are discussed in the story about Sheryl and Roger in Chapter 3.

2. Rehearse.

Review the major concerns you have together before you go to the appointment. It will enable you to anticipate possible answers and to think of further questions.

3. If you can, schedule more than one visit.

Dr. Gabriel Hortobagyi's clinic treats more breast cancer patients than any one facility in the world. Time is crucial in this busy clinic, so Dr. Hortobagyi recommends scheduling two short visits before treatment starts. "I respect families who want to use our time in a way that will be most beneficial to them and to me," he says.

Dr. Eugene Carlton explains why this system works well: "If it's the first time I tell a family about the cancer, I assume they will be in shock. Anything else I say will be wiped out. By the second visit, they've read about what I've told them and organized their questions.

"Then we sit down and go over the treatment plan. They may agree to it, they may go for a second opinion, or they may go home to think about it and schedule a time to talk by phone."

Although second visits can be conducted over the phone, Dr. Carlton advises, "If you still have questions that you want answered in person, call your doctor and say, 'We have additional questions. I would like an appointment to concentrate on them.' If the doctor refuses, you should get another doctor."

4. Confirm all doctors' appointments.

Many doctors, especially surgeons, have last-minute changes in their schedules. Although many offices will try to contact you to change your appointment before you leave, some will not. It is in your best interest to confirm your appointment an hour before you leave the house. If your appointment is the first in the morning, then call at five o'clock the afternoon before to confirm.

BIZARRO   By DAN PIRARO

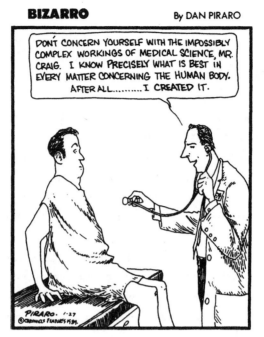

5. Ask the patient if it would help if she were fully clothed at the beginning of the appointment.

Patients can request to start their first visit while dressed. "This may decrease feelings of embarrassment and intimidation," says psychiatrist Dr. Alan Valentine.

6. Establish how you will address each other.

Some patients feel that having their doctor call them by their last name maintains a level of professionalism in their relationship. They are offended if the doctor refers to them by their first name. They would never consider calling a doctor by his or her first name.

I have always been more at ease being on a first-name basis with doctors. Using last names seems to inject too much distance and sometimes a bit of coldness. You and your loved one have to decide what is most comfortable. Make your preference known to the doctor if you have one.

7. If you get confused, stop the doctor and ask him to clarify.

Dr. Hortobagyi advises you to say, "Look, we've been talking for fifteen minutes. I know you are trying to do your best, but this is hard for me to comprehend. I will understand better if you compare it to how a car works, or use a diagram or plastic model."

8. Ask the doctor to define any term you don't understand.

"Tell your doctor that he is speaking with a vocabulary you don't understand," says Richard Theriault in an article in the M. D. Anderson *Network* Newsletter. "Don't be embarrassed or bashful about not knowing what everything means. A lot of people come in afraid to ask questions because they think it will be a 'dumb question' or so insignificant that they can't possibly bring it up. Any concerns and questions are important, and they need to be discussed."

9. If you've heard too much for one day, say so.

Unless you stop the doctor, she won't know when you are overwhelmed. When you have heard enough for one day, Dr. Hortobagyi suggests you tell her, "I'm on information overload. Can we stop here and schedule another time to continue?"

Most doctors want you to understand what they are telling you. Dr. Hortobagyi adds, "Nothing is worse than doing everything you can to explain something to a family and then finding out that they missed some or a lot of important information, and that this gap led to a misunderstanding or confusion. This can be avoided if families are honest with their doctors."

10. Use appointment time wisely.

I asked one doctor why some patients walk away frustrated from doctors' appointments. He gave me one reason: "Often people come with a tape recorder, a companion, and a list of questions. Then halfway through our discussion they get off the subject. They talk about a neighbor or a relative. They want to tell me this other patient's entire story."

Do not spend your visit talking about the patient you just met in the waiting room or about other people with similar illnesses. It takes too long to explain and their story may not be relevant to yours.

Suppose someone has told you about the side effects of a drug your loved one is taking or some other problem. When you ask about it, focus on how it could affect your loved one. Say, "We've heard this could be a side effect. Is that true?" Or: "This is what we're worried about."

11. Be assertive.

Families who state their questions and concerns clearly, in a brief, organized, concise manner will have a better chance of getting their needs met. Whenever a problem is still not resolved, ask the doctor to explain why.

If a doctor says he can't manage a symptom, encourage the patient to ask him for a referral. It may be that no one can. For example, as Dr. Valentine cautions, "Symptoms like insomnia are very difficult to treat in some patients." But ask for another opinion anyway.

When pain cannot be controlled, ask to see a pain specialist. If your doctor can't or won't refer you to one himself, call the National Chronic Pain Outreach Association (301-652-4948, or on the Internet at http://neurosurgery.mgh.harvard.edu/ncpainoa.htm). Director Doug Ventura explains that the NCPOA provides referrals to member health professionals and medical facilities nationwide, maintains a registry of chronic pain support groups, and publishes brochures and a quarterly newsletter, *Lifeline*, which offers practical techniques for coping with pain. Another organization that provides lists of support groups is the American Chronic Pain Association (916-632-0922, or at www.theacpa.org).

Mental Health Association agencies can also be of help. At Cancer Counseling our psychiatrists and psychologists work with patients who have problems such as pain, depression, and insomnia. If you go to an outside agency about symptoms, the professionals there should always coordinate any care they provide with the patient's doctor.

Chronic pain can affect every area of a patient's life in a negative way. It can affect sleep, moods, concentration, and the ability to perform even seemingly simple tasks. Treating cancer pain is such a global problem that the World Health Organization has urged every nation to establish a pain policy. If your doctor cannot help your loved one, look for a doctor who can. It may take many visits before the pain can be managed, but reducing it is vital to the patient's well-being and yours.

12. Rephrase unanswered questions.

"She's not sleeping at night. Is there something you can treat her insomnia with?"

"She feels tired all day. What can we do?"

"She's exhausted most of the time because she isn't getting any rest. Is there something to help her sleep?"

Sometimes the doctor just didn't hear you or was distracted. Other times he did hear you and responded, but you didn't understand the answer or want to hear it.

One physician said, "Families think if they ask me the same question five different ways, I'll change my mind. It's hard on them. If they feel they aren't getting their questions answered, I recommend they bring along a second family member or a hospital social worker or a nurse practitioner. They may discover they just don't like the answers. Or maybe I don't understand their questions. Another 'ear' can help clear up this problem."

13. Use a third set of ears.

If you are having problems understanding or communicating with the physician, ask if a social worker, nurse practitioner, or oncology nurse practitioner can act as a "third set of ears." When patients and family members alike are nervous and uncomfortable, it may be difficult to concentrate or take notes.

"Third ears" should only take notes—they should not give advice. Although they may assist you in formulating questions that arise out of the meeting, they should never try to influence a patient in any way about a treatment decision.

I would not recommend using a third ear unless you have exhausted all other ways of understanding your doctors and the patient doesn't want to use a tape recorder. Complications can arise when well-meaning outsiders are included in confidential family-doctor meetings.

14. Discuss alternative treatments without lecturing.

Many physicians have strong opinions about alternative treatments. "It doesn't matter what I think," one doctor pointed out. "If I can't offer it, then it's a waste of time to have a long discussion about it.

"If patients come to me, they need to focus on what I have to offer them. They can ask my opinion about a treatment, but then they must accept it for what it's worth and get back to discussing how I can help them. Some families want to spend an entire visit arguing about a drug like laetrile that I can't even give them."

Another doctor agreed. "I'd rather patients advised me of their interests," he added. "When I've thought an alternative therapy was viable, I've called the researchers and investigated. If it was something that could help, I encouraged families to look into it further. I've also assisted them in enrolling in studies, including some administered by my colleagues in other countries." Let your doctor and pharmacist know about the over-the-counter and herbal supplements you are taking to ensure you don't experience adverse reactions.

15. Take notes and/or tape-record the visit.

Offer to take notes at doctors' appointments so the patient can concentrate on the doctor. Even if you take notes, use a tape recorder too. The notes will help you know which sections to play back later. The patient may want to play the tape for family members who couldn't be present, such as an out-of-town spouse or an adult child who is a primary caregiver. The tape will also be invaluable for future reference and to clear up any misunderstandings. After the appointment, play back the tape while the meeting is fresh in your mind. This will help clarify unfamiliar terms or comments in your notes.

16. Repeat the instructions at the end of the visit.

Before you leave, make sure you have understood the instructions correctly by repeating them back to your doctor. Also, ask the doctor when is the best time to call if you get home and realize you have more questions.

17. After the appointment, review the instructions and information.

Verbalizing what you have heard clarifies it. You will both develop a clearer understanding of what you have been told, and talking together can generate additional questions to ask later.

18. Don't rush. Don't push.

Dr. Hortobagyi warns, "No one should feel rushed about making a decision about a treatment, especially at the beginning."

Every doctor I interviewed agreed with him. Yet they had different ideas about how long it should take to make a decision. The average time they recommended was two weeks. Some families need more time to do research and get second and third opinions, but usually a two-to-three-week delay in starting treatment will not lessen the effectiveness of treatment. Ask your doctor to make sure your loved one's situation is no exception. Taking time in the beginning can become important later, because it is vital that patients feel comfortable with their final decision about treatment.

As a caregiver, do not push a patient into making this decision. You will only create resentment. If something goes wrong later, you could have problems with yourself (guilt) and with the patient (anger and resentment).

19. Try to be a sounding board.

While the patient is making the decision, you can act as a sounding board by pointing out alternatives. Do not urge the patient to undergo a treatment he opposes. This is another fine line you will have to walk.

When my father called me in 1993 and told me about the care my mother was getting, I got furious. So I probably was not a very good sounding board for him. Fortunately, my parents were already looking for alternatives.

My mother's first doctors thought her tumor was inoperable. Even when they made adjustments in their prognosis, they had no immediate plans of operating. Meanwhile I referred her to Memorial Sloan-Kettering, where she was operated on within two weeks. Fortunately, the fast-growing tumor had not spread. Had she waited much longer, she would not have survived.

This man tried to act as the advocate for his grandmother against her wishes: "My mother and I started to push my grandmother into getting another opinion before she started her chemotherapy. However, I could tell she liked the doctor she was seeing. After a few attempts to get her to see someone else, I told my mother we should both back off and just pray my grandmother was in good hands.

"That was four years ago. Today my grandmother is cancer free. What if we had pushed her into seeing another doctor and there were complications, or the results weren't as good?"

20. Use statistics as guidelines, not as personal predictions.

Kevin, the thirty-one-year-old husband of a patient, learned that his wife had only a five percent chance of surviving. "We gave up all hope," he says. "Then our doctor reminded us about the five percent that do survive. Why couldn't she be one of them?"

Judith, a thirty-two-year-old widow, holds another view of statistics. "Our doctor always focused on the fifty percent that survived," she says. "So we never even considered the possibility that my husband wasn't going to make it. I'm still angry at how the doctor's overly positive attitude affected us. He never prepared us for what could go wrong. My husband's gone now. I've never been this angry. I feel like we were so busy fighting the disease, we never focused on living or preparing for a future without him. I have four kids, an overdue mortgage, and an attic full of files that I don't have a clue about handling."

Statistics are guidelines, not predictions. Their numbers include patients who have other illnesses and contributing factors that your loved one may not have. On the other hand, a patient with a twenty percent chance of survival is in a serious situation. Eighty percent of the patients with the same diagnosis do not survive. These patients ought to organize affairs as best they can, but then they should focus on enjoying and appreciating whatever time they have.

All of us should do this. In one of my support groups the patients and spouses filled out their wills, living wills, and durable powers of attorney, and they made sure their finances were organized. If the situation is getting worse and the patient says, "I don't like the statistics. I want to stop treatment. I'd rather enjoy what time I do have," then respect his wishes. Pushing for a two percent cure when the patient does not agree is not supporting him.

21. Discuss second opinions.

Jo Ann Ward, director of CIS of Texas and Oklahoma, is a strong believer in getting a second opinion. Not only does she recommend second opinions to CIS callers, she obtained one for a family member's diagnosis. "My father was diagnosed with a rare form of cancer that would have required major facial surgery and recovery.

"Like many people of his generation, he was reluctant to tell his doctor he wanted a second opinion. But I kept trying to convince him to get one.

"I admit I finally resorted to a father-daughter emotional ploy. I said that with all my knowledge about cancer and its treatment, I'd never forgive myself if we didn't do everything possible to make sure he had the right diagnosis.

"He agreed to come to M. D. Anderson for a second opinion. For us it was a blessing—his true diagnosis was completely different from what he had first been told.

"Then he made his decision about treatment, one that was hard for me. He chose to not have life-prolonging treatment. But it was his decision and my turn to honor his wishes. During his last months he enjoyed a quality of life that was the best possible, and he avoided a useless, disfiguring surgery.

"So if you're thinking about getting a second opinion, you'll probably be glad if you follow through."

Justin went to four major cancer centers to decide whether chemotherapy or surgery would be the better treatment for his tumor. The opinions he received differed so widely that he and his wife, Annie, were frustrated every time they came to my group.

I asked him to sit down and decide what he wanted to do. A week later he answered, "This is what I want to do. I want it out. I want the surgery. I'll do the other stuff later. The problem is, no one wants to operate first."

I encouraged him to ask two of the cancer centers to consult with each other. They had a meeting and decided they would do as Justin wanted. As soon as the operation was over, his wife called me. "They just finished, and I'm calling to thank you. They found a second tumor that would have caused damage to his lungs. If they hadn't gone in today, he would have died in a matter of months."

Before your loved one embarks on any treatment, he ought to get a second opinion. Dr. Hortobagyi advises you to "take the time in the beginning to make sure about the therapy. Once we start a protocol, it's more effective if we do it according to a schedule." Numerous factors contribute to establishing this schedule. It is better for both the patient and the physician if the patient evaluates all his options be-fore the doctor develops the treatment plan.

Why else should you get a second opinion?

- The patient can reassure herself that she has heard more than one alternative and has done everything she can.
- It can prevent her from undergoing a treatment that may make no difference to her health but will destroy the quality of her life.
- The patient may find a doctor who better suits his needs.
- The patient will be reassured that other doctors agree with the treatment plan and the alternatives are not acceptable.
- The patient will understand the risks better.
- A patient who undergoes certain treatments may be precluded from doing others later. If tissue is damaged by radiation, for ex-ample, surgery may no longer be an option.
- It's worth every penny. "Most insurance companies provide re-imbursement for second opinions and sometimes even third opinions," Dr. Eugene Carlton explains. "Even if they don't, it is absolutely worth the money and the time to go." Second opinions are less expensive—financially, emotionally, and phys-ically—than ill-advised treatments.
- An outsider will review the whole picture.

Dr. Carlton advises obtaining a complete workup from someone who specializes in that affected part of the body. "They have a broad view of the disease, of side effects, and of the most effective treat-ment. They don't have a bias toward an expertise—surgery, radiation, or chemotherapy."

The specialists he recommends practice in these areas: pulmonary, neurosurgery, urology, gynecology, orthopedics, hematology, medical oncology, or breast cancer. You can get names of specialists by using the Resources section.

"Whenever possible, try to go to a teaching hospital or major medical center, where a multidisciplinary approach is usually offered." A team of doctors will review the patient's individualized case in a meeting called a consult.

When a patient and a loved one have to make an especially difficult decision, they can request that an outsider (a medical ethicist or the family physician) attend the consult on the patient's behalf.

A final reason to get a second opinion is to get help devising a plan. Many physicians I have worked with send patients to a major medical school or cancer center for a second opinion. One New Jersey doctor said, "I didn't want to treat Mr. Brady until someone at a major medical center had given us another opinion. At first I worked with them on a plan for therapy. A few years later I sent Mr. Brady to the Mayo Clinic to participate in an experimental treatment. Despite his original prognosis, which was poor, he is alive today. It's partly because his chemotherapy protocols were devised by colleagues from different places who knew how to work together."

Your loved one may be interested in obtaining a second opinion but may not be willing to travel to another medical center or medical school. In this case, enlist the help of the primary doctor. She can send records, slides, and X rays to the center, then work with the center to develop a plan that can be administered close to home.

Dr. Hortobagyi cautions: "Patients should be prepared, when seeking a second opinion, that it might be different from the first opinion. In fact, a third opinion might be different from the first and second. That's why it's important to have a physician you trust, one with whom you can discuss all three opinions, to explain the differences and help you reach a decision."

When to Leave a Doctor

Leaving a doctor is completely up to the patient. She, more than anyone else, has to be comfortable with the medical care she is receiving. Most health care professionals believe patients should never go to a doctor with whom they feel uncomfortable. I agree, to a point.

A patient of mine said she really didn't like her surgeon that much. Her husband did not like him either, and her social worker advised going to someone else. But the patient was about to have a very complicated surgery. "I trusted this doctor more than anyone in the world to operate," she said.

Since the doctor believed she'd need only one procedure, she decided to tolerate his bedside manner in the light of his skills and reputation. Her unconditional faith in him was a vital part of her ability to cope with the possibility that she might not survive the operation. Knowing he was performing the surgery enabled her to have a positive attitude. Trusting a doctor is as important as liking him—although the latter helps.

To this woman's surprise, the doctor was much warmer on follow-up visits. Even if he had not been, however, she could have gone to someone else for her quarterly checkups.

Consider leaving your doctor if he:

- consistently ignores your questions
- doesn't listen to your concerns
- is rude
- refuses to explain terms in a way you can understand
- refuses to give you any hope. The hope need not be for a cure—it can be for good care, or to keep the patient comfortable and pain free, or to maximize the quality of life.
- refuses to have a meeting just to answer your questions
- refuses to refer you for a second opinion
- just doesn't make the patient feel comfortable

If the patient doesn't trust the doctor or have faith in him, then most experts would encourage him to find another doctor. A patient's trust, comfort, and respect are essential to a good doctor-patient relationship.

Other Resources

NURSES

When my mother checked in at Sloan-Kettering, no beds were available on the floor for lung cancer patients. So they assigned her to a room in the part of the hospital reserved for colon cancer patients. One of the nurses, Barb, went out of her way to take care of my mother. After my mother's surgery she was moved to the lung cancer floor. As my husband and I were visiting, Barb poked her head in: "I just wanted to see how you are doing. Don't let me interrupt." But we all wanted her to interrupt. She reminded us of that other room, that other place, the place my mother was the night we did not know whether she would live or die. It was as though Barb had stepped out of that place, that world, as my mother had, and entered this one.

Barb sat on the corner of my mother's bed and explained to us her plans for what was left of the long Memorial Day weekend. "No, I don't have a boyfriend at the moment, but I am working on it." She laughed. "I do have a cat, and my brother's here." I watched her converse with my mother like an old friend, my mother absorbed in every word Barb spoke. My mother now belonged to a part of Barb's world, and only she and Barb could understand where my mother had just been, the operation she had endured. Only they could really appreciate the magnitude of what my mother had just survived.

When I was six months pregnant, I spent two weeks in the hospital trying to save my son's life. Every nurse I met was compassionate and went out of her way to make me feel that I was not alone. And when my son died, a nurse from another floor, one who usually dealt with delivering healthy babies, came into the room, sat on the bed, and said, "Are you okay?" I shook my head, and then she whispered, "I will just stay here as long as you need me." She was exactly what I needed. There are bad nurses, nastier than the wicked witch. But if you are assertive rather than aggressive, and if you are courteous, kind, and interject humor occasionally, a nurse will appreciate your consideration. She may even become one of your greatest allies.

A nurse who takes the patient or you under her wing makes a tremendous difference in a hospital stay. Most nurses are eager to help, although I am not sure how many would track down a patient that they had met only for a brief moment, one who was no longer theirs.

Nurses in doctors' offices are another invaluable resource. One woman said, "We love our doctor, but we just can't understand everything he says when we are with him. We don't expect him to meet all of our needs. So whenever we need anything explained, be it medication, side effects, or symptoms, we call Greta, his nurse. She always answers our questions or gets answers from the doctor herself. She has this way of making us feel like we can handle whatever problems we are having. When we needed to switch over to hospice, she checked in periodically to see how we were doing. I knew she was still there to answer any questions I had or to just listen if I needed to talk. She always managed to point us in the right direction and to make us feel that she was right there beside us. The last time I saw her was at my husband's funeral, quietly standing behind me. She still calls. She still checks in. She even sends Christmas cards."

STAFF PSYCHIATRISTS

Staff psychiatrists are an auxiliary service you may not need. In some circumstances, though, it becomes imperative that you use one. Dr. Valentine suggests, "A psychiatric evaluation is indicated if a patient is suicidal or severely depressed. An evaluation can be useful for milder depression and for other problems, including anxiety, insomnia, and memory loss."

If you are in the room when the psychiatrist arrives to see the patient, let him conduct the visit without your interference. "When the psychiatrist or any doctor comes into the room," Dr. Valentine adds, "unless the patient is incoherent, caregivers should not answer for him or her. Let doctors ask the questions. Let patients answer them. This enables the physician to make an assessment.

"If a patient informs you he doesn't trust his memory because of the medication, tell the doctor. As a caregiver, you should still not answer for the patient unless the doctor directs the question to you."

SOCIAL WORKERS

Allison Stovall describes the role of hospital social workers: "Families in the hospital are highly dependent on the staff for everything. They feel beholden to them. Social workers can help patients and families gain some semblance of control in this situation. They can teach them how to access resources in the hospital system. They'll help them formulate their questions and make requests to the staff for what they need during the stay.

"Social workers will help them cope with the changes they encounter and prepare them for what is going to happen before a crisis occurs. We can also act as facilitators with people they may not be comfortable with."

I asked for Jean, a social worker, to see my mother at Sloan-Kettering so that she could have someone to call if she had problems adjusting when she went home. My father heard about my request, and said to me, "She's going to kill you. She doesn't want to talk to a counselor now."

If you ask my mother who has helped her the most over the past four years, Jean will be among the names she gives. Once she said: "Jean understands me and how I feel. She always gives me something to hold on to, something to think about."

Your loved one doesn't have to be exhibiting any problems to benefit from connecting with a social worker. Even if they meet in person only once, it gives the patient a face to associate with a name. If she ever needs someone, she'll have a person she can call.

PATIENT ADVOCATES

Dr. Donna Copeland, the child psychologist introduced in Chapter 9, advises families to find someone on staff who can act as their advocate. It may be the designated hospital advocate, but it can also be a nurse, an intern, a chaplain, a psychologist, or a psychiatrist. "An advocate can teach the patient and the family to identify their needs and to be assertive enough to speak out for themselves," says Dr. Copeland. An advocate can assist you with problems related to hospital care, be it the nurse you are having problems with or the temperature of the food.

CHAPLAINS

Steve Thorney, a chaplain in the Texas Medical Center, plays a liaison role. "A family who is having trouble with the staff or with each other can use me as a resource. I'll sit with them and help them resolve their issues." Most hospital chaplains have extensive experience working with serious medical problems.

When I led a support group with Steve, I was always impressed with his sensitivity toward families. For six years my patients, of all denominations, had raved about another chaplain, Sister Alice Potts. They would say, "There is no one like her." Upon meeting her, I knew why: She has a gift with patients that few can match. If you can find a Sister Alice or a Steve Thorney, someone who is sensitive to your needs and beliefs, they can hold your hand, as well as the patient's, and guide you through this ordeal.

You may be uncomfortable, however, when a chaplain, volunteer, or social worker enters the hospital room unannounced. Feel free to say, "I appreciate your interest, but I need to be alone." If you do decide to use a chaplain, John Stelling, conference chair of the 1995 M. D. Anderson Outpatient Ministry conference, recommends that you ask the chaplain about his credentials and the extent of his experience with families coping with your present issues.

VOLUNTEERS

A volunteer can keep a hospitalized patient company, comfort you when you feel alone, and provide practical assistance to you and the patient. Volunteers also provide numerous household services when the patient is homebound. They will accompany and sometimes drive patients to doctors' visits, take them on walks, baby-sit if you need to go somewhere, and attend to the patient's physical and emotional needs. Call the hospital volunteer department or your senior center, congregation, local American Cancer Society, or United Way to ask about how volunteers can help care for your loved one.

The services and suggestions in this chapter are meant to make your life easier as well as the patient's. However, you may not be interested in meeting with hospital staff people. One patient who went to a hospital for a second opinion told me that before she even saw the doctor, nurses and social workers and chaplains came to meet with her. She did not want to talk to anybody but her doctor and was quite upset at having to tell each person that she didn't want to talk. At another time she might have been interested in meeting them, but during this visit their presence was extremely upsetting. If you do not want to talk to hospital staff, it is perfectly okay. Upon checking in, tell the receptionist, "For the time being we would not like to see anyone but our doctor and her nurses. If you have other people such as chaplains or social workers, could you please give us their cards and we will contact them on our own?" Feel free to call them later, even after the patient has been released.

While my mother was in the hospital that Memorial Day weekend, we greatly appreciated most of the hospital staff. They made our worst nightmare as positive as it could be. But another aspect of her stay, one that only Barb, the nurse, mentioned, was the overriding fact that this was a holiday, the beginning of summer, the end of a long hard winter. It was a holiday unlike any we had known before.

All of our holidays were forever changed when cancer swept into our lives, as yours will be. The next chapter will provide ways for you to negotiate these marks on your calendar—days filled with meaning, expectations, hopes, and fears.

Chapter 13

Making Holidays Meaningful

Right before Thanksgiving, my mother was rushed to the hospital for an emergency appendectomy. Fifteen hundred miles away, I sat by the phone in the dark for hours, imagining what life would be like without her, praying that she would make it to Thanksgiving, to tomorrow. She did, but that Christmas was tinged with relief and fear. She was tired, more so than I'd ever seen her. Every move seemed an effort. By Mother's Day she still was not feeling well, but I was so busy rejoicing that I still had another Mother's Day that I did not even notice what must have been cleverly couched beneath her announcement, "I've quit smoking." But it wasn't the smoking she had to escape—it was asbestos and she already knew it. She didn't say a word to me. And then my dad called, saying she had lung cancer. Within days she was scheduled for surgery on Memorial Day weekend. It changed every single holiday we have had since.

Take New Year's Eve, for example, the one after my mother's surgery. It was not exactly what we had expected. Although I relished the dinner conversation and my mother's smiles, and although I loved dancing with my father, my pregnant belly barely hidden by the loose-fitting sequined top, the evening was nevertheless marred. I couldn't help but notice the shadows of pain that slid across my mother's eyes.

And then last year, we were so sure this would be the New Year's when we would really celebrate. We arranged for a baby-sitter. We had the tuxes, the sequined dresses, the Country Club reservations.

On December thirtieth my mother called. "Do you really want to go tomorrow night?" she asked.

"Why?" I replied.

"Well," she said, "we had a thought. What would you think about ordering pizza and spending a cozy night here? We can all get dressed up in the tuxes and dresses and drink champagne and watch the ball drop on TV."

I stumbled for a minute, visualizing my mother at the club, dancing in my father's arms, all dressed up, laughing. "Forget the tuxes," I said. "We'll come casual. When do you want us?"

The next night, there we were, all of us curled up on their long, dark green couch, and there was pizza and our family friend Billy. We talked until the Times Square ball dropped, ate the absolutely delicious pizza, and had the finest New Year's ever.

We had endured a lot, all of us: Billy's wife's death a few years before, the death of my son, my grandmother's recent death, my mother's cancer, and her constant battle with pain. But that night for a few short hours, it was all forgotten. Every moment was filled with a sense of celebration and joy. Holidays, for us, have been filled with expectations and disappointments, with fears and pain and memories, but in those few hours, that holiday became a celebration, a victory over all we had overcome. I left with a feeling of renewal about all we could conquer in the future. And never once, as I had done on so many other holidays, did I wonder whether my mother would be with us for the next one. I was enjoying the moment and thanking God she was here for this one.

Holidays are milestones. As each one comes into view, memories of those gone by reemerge. We reevaluate where we are, where we came from, and where we are going.

Holidays are to be celebrated, but when an illness strikes, they take on a new meaning—often not a positive one. But you can't stop them from coming or ignore them. The world around us announces them with Easter baskets in the supermarket, Santa Clauses on the street, parking lots filled with trees, catalogs in the mail, and specials on TV.

Every November the people in my support groups would wrestle with their feelings about the holidays. And just as they overcame the challenges of the fall and winter festivities, another set of holidays would emerge—Valentine's Day, Easter, and Father's and Mother's Days. Once again they would be forced to focus on ways to cope. These events were hardest on my group members who expected too much of themselves, and on those whose loved ones weren't feeling well or were dying, or whose family members made too many demands.

Dylan, a cancer patient, had young children. A few weeks before Thanksgiving, his wife, Nicole, said to the group, "While the rest of the world is making plans to celebrate, we are praying Dylan will just wake up that morning." Vacillating between terror and hope, she added, "It's his favorite holiday. I just know he'll survive. But how do I deal with this? How do I get my kids through?"

When Jordy's parents wanted him and his wife, Christine, to come for Hanukkah, she said to her husband, "I know your parents have been really good to us since you've been ill, and I realize how much they want us to go there for Hanukkah. But I just can't deal with the holiday rush, the airports, the cabs, the packing. What do you think about visiting them in January?"

Jordy said, "I don't know. I want to go, but I understand how you feel. And now that I'm doing so well, we will have lots of holidays together."

Christine felt a stab of guilt. What if the cancer came back? What if it was worse next time? What if something happened to his parents? What if... "Okay, we'll go," she announced. They did go.

Five years later, Christine recalled that "it took me months to recover from that trip. Before we even got on the plane, I was exhausted from caring for Jordy and my daughter, Sabrina. Having to be in his parents' home, and having his mother hover over him and me, was more than I could handle. And to make it worse, his father was ill, so we spent six days listening to the details of his ailments. Any other time I might have been more compassionate, but this was the one holiday I just wanted to celebrate with Jordy and my newborn daughter."

Terrance's children called just about every day to talk about their holiday plans. The entire family was going to meet in Maine to share Christmas. His wife, Mira, enjoyed the excitement, but Terrance knew she was pushing herself pretty hard, given that she was in the middle of radiation treatment. Whenever the couple came to the support group, the first thing Mira always talked about was the Christmas trip. Terrance, for his part, just couldn't picture making the long journey north. Finally, Mira decided the trip was really too much—greatly to his relief. They saw their children in January and enjoyed them more than they ever would have had they gone during the holidays.

Guidelines for Holidays

1. You can't change the circumstances, but you can decide how to spend a holiday.

If you used to write cards and now you don't want to, don't do it. If you used to send a family letter but now you just can't type it, forget it this year. If you always shopped months in advance and now you don't even know what month it is, then give up the shopping.

Whatever causes you and your loved one stress ought to be reevaluated. Holidays are very difficult, and you don't need the burden of maintaining a tradition this year. If you have kids, find other ways to have fun with them. Go to the movies, order in pizza, see a show, have friends cook that dinner they have been offering to cook. You can keep the holiday—just throw out the old tradition and try another one this year. If you are completely exhausted, your kids aren't going to enjoy it anyway.

This holiday you may be wondering whether it is the last you will have with your loved one, no matter how healthy he is. Think about ways to celebrate your lives together, ways you will both really appreciate. What would leave you feeling like it was a good holiday? If you have kids, have a family meeting (described in Chapter 10) and ask them to brainstorm ways to celebrate. You may be surprised at how imaginative they can be.

2. Decide what you want.

Ask yourself the following questions, and write the answers in your journal or notebook.

- What is your favorite ritual?
- What is your least favorite?
- Which rituals would you like to change?
- Which customs do your children look forward to?
- What do you want to do this holiday?
- What is your fondest memory of this holiday?
- If you could do anything you wished, within reason, how would you celebrate this holiday?

Ask your loved one the same questions, and write them down too.

3. Choose ways to celebrate that make you and your loved one feel good.

Sometimes we forget the true meaning of holidays. They are to be enjoyed and spent with people we care about. It's difficult to remember if we become caught up in other people's perceptions about how to celebrate, or if we spend them with relatives whose company we don't enjoy.

Holidays usually include rituals that can bring people together, create excitement, and provide continuity. The rituals are important, but now you may need or want to change them. The rituals you create can be as meaningful as the ones you are about to leave behind.

You can also keep old traditions by mixing them with new, more suitable ones. Don't be afraid of interjecting your wishes into a celebration—you'll bring a positive atmosphere to it. By including children, friends, and family in the process of altering traditions, you'll create a feeling of belonging and make change easier for them.

4. Make changes.

Next, think about the changes you can make. Can you go to your brother's home for another holiday, when there's less pressure, instead of for Passover? Better yet, can you postpone visiting until after any holiday?

Four years ago Beverly was recovering from chemotherapy when Passover crept up on her calendar. Her husband, Murray, didn't want them to spend the holiday with her family, since they always fought and complained when they got together.

Murray wanted to be with people who would make Beverly feel peaceful, positive, and welcome. Sandra and Andy Kaplan, their close friends, had invited them to spend the holiday with them. They had kids the same age as Murray and Beverly's.

Murray accepted the Kaplans' invitation. He and Beverly appeased their families by scheduling visits with them after the holidays. As Beverly's son explained, "Passover is fun since we started going to the Kaplans'. Mom is relaxed, and Dad enjoys himself. It brings us closer as a family, a much happier family than we were when we felt trapped entertaining people who weren't grateful to be together."

Sometimes you can spend the holiday with the same people but change the way you spend it. Robert, whom you met in Chapter 1, describes the change his family made: "My sister suggested we go around the table and tell each other what we were thankful for. I thought it was ridiculous. We always enjoyed Thanksgiving—now she wanted to turn our easy conversation into something too personal.

"It was amazing. Once you took the time to reflect, you realized how many blessings you were thankful for. Slightly altering a tradition can make it take on a whole new meaning. It transformed the proverbial turkey dinner into an evening to cherish."

5. If a new tradition doesn't work, you can change it next year.

"I dragged the darn tree all the way through the front yard," complains Greg, who was recovering from cancer surgery. "I trudged into the basement and yanked out the cartons of tangled lights. No one really had an interest in decorating. We usually go to my wife's parents', but I wasn't up to it last year, so we decided to have Christmas alone and do it ourselves.

"The kids screamed. The lights got tangled around my wife's cat, which was the only entertaining part of the night. When the lights finally did get set up, I turned them on, and they proceeded to short out, one at a time. A few survivors blinked pathetically at me. It was the worst Christmas ever.

"This year I was in the middle of pulling out the carton when I asked my wife if we really needed to go through the same fiasco as last year. I was undergoing radiation, and I just wasn't ready for another holiday like that one. She agreed to make another change. We went out and bought one of those three-foot trees—the cheap plastic green kind."

His wife tells how much better the celebration went. "My husband decorated it with one strand of white lights, put our favorite ornament on top, then placed it in the center of the living room. Now you might think, 'Those poor pathetic people,' but it was such a relief not to have to deal with decorating a tree.

"The night we usually set aside for decorating, we decided to go for a ride. Piling into my husband's truck, with jugs of warm apple cider and our three kids, we toured the homes in the valley. One after another, each street welcomed us with its vast intricate decorations. As these incredible displays unfolded, our pain melted away. As our ten-month-old pointed and tried his best to describe these sights, we burst out laughing.

"Changing our plans freed us from the shackles of tradition. We focused on what was important—each other."

Approach a new tradition as an adventure, with your sense of humor in hand. Realize ahead of time that it may not work. At least you had the courage to try something new—you can always change the plans again next year.

6. Write down your needs ahead of time.

Make a list of at least ten projects you think you have to complete for this holiday season. Now go back through the list and cross off any items that you will definitely not get to or you can live without. Maybe you hate baking—cross it off. Replace it with "Buy breads, cakes, or cookies from the bakery or gourmet shop."

7. Keep a plan if you can, even if others no longer want to.

If you decide you want to attend a scheduled event but other family members have changed their minds, go anyway. It's okay to go alone.

"I was getting ready for an Easter celebration with good friends," explains Terry. "These people had been kind to me over the years. I always found their company, and that of their relatives, uplifting.

"The night of the party, I walked into the living room. My husband was sprawled on the couch, popcorn in one hand, flipper in the other. He wasn't moving. I stormed back into our room. How could he do this? He'd said he was having a good day. He'd said he wanted to go. He undermines everything, I thought, using the cancer as an excuse. When are we going to find time to enjoy ourselves?

"Then I eased into my chair, looked in the mirror, and said, 'But I want to go.' Guilt slapped me in the face. 'You can't go—leave him behind. How dare you? What do you think you're doing?' I sat up. 'Taking care of me.'

"Fortunately, before I went in and raised holy hell, I calmed down somewhat. Then I went back to him and said, 'Honey, I really want to do this, I need to do this. I want to be part of the celebration, and I understand fully that you may not want to. Do you mind if I go alone?'

"I waited for his diatribe: 'How could you? You're selfish! What about me?' Instead he pulled me toward him and stroked my hair and said, 'I wish you would go. I don't want you to miss the party, but right now I need some time alone. I'm just not up to socializing. Anyway, there's a movie I want to watch.'

"When I arrived back home, he was eager to hear about our friends. There wasn't a hint of resentment in his tone—only admiration that I had gone alone."

This crisis could have turned out quite differently. An explosion could have followed, and weeks of repercussions. They never happened. Terry had the courage to go alone but didn't make her husband feel guilty for staying home.

8. Give special gifts.

- Give heirlooms, other personal treasures, or a letter describing the contributions the person has made in your life or the fond memories you have of her.
- Take the family to a comedy, musical, or play.
- Get ideas for gift certificates from Chapter 5.
- Rent a Santa or Easter bunny to entertain kids for an hour.
- Drop off a bottle of champagne wrapped in silver or gold paper with a personal note, sending your best wishes for a happy holiday, birthday, or anniversary. Include two champagne glasses, cheeses, and crackers.
- Give a membership to a nearby zoo, museum, playhouse, or exercise club.
- Buy a gift from a charity event, antique show, or home or jewelry exhibits.
- Make a home movie, and give it as a gift.
- Buy a meaningful but generic gift. If you have found bath oils

you love, frames you like, or books you think are great, buy extras and keep them stored for special occasions to avoid last-minute shopping.

- Make up a personalized photo album of your family. It will be especially treasured by a grandparent.
- Give a family photo already framed.

9. Enjoy other aspects of the holiday besides gifts.

- Spend an evening watching home videos or going through family albums.
- Read a Christmas book together.
- Listen to music or sing together.
- Write your spouse or the patient a love letter or a poem.
- Take a long walk, either outside or in a mall.
- Contact a friend who you know will be alone, and invite her over for Chinese food, pizza, or a meal taken out from a local restaurant.
- Go to an upbeat movie.
- Rent movies like *Santa Claus,* Bill Murray's *Scrooge,* or any of Disney's animated cartoons.
- Sit by a skating rink and watch the kids enjoy themselves, or take your loved one skating if he can.
- Go away—take the family to a cabin for fishing, hunting, or cross-country skiing.
- Ask the grandparents to share stories about how they spent the holidays as children.
- Smile more, and thank anyone who is courteous or kind.

People thrive on recognition. Compliment your kids, spouse, or friends on a job well done or an act of kindness or any other contribution they make toward the holiday.

10. Share responsibilities.

If you have adult kids you entertain every year, ask them *what* they want to contribute to the holiday this year, not *if* they want to help out.

When you delegate something, let it go. It doesn't have to be done perfectly. Be grateful for the help instead of critical of the quality.

If the patient or the caregiver is your host, don't go to him with complaints. Handle whatever crisis occurs so he will be free to enjoy the holiday without any unnecessary burdens.

11. Set your limits.

This is the year to do what you want to do for the holidays. Make plans to do only things that you have an interest in doing. If you don't want to attend an event, let your friends and family know in advance. Say, "I'm sorry, but I won't be able to do that this year. Please check with me next year, when my circumstances might be different."

If you're not sure about an invitation, accept it conditionally: "We'd really like to come, but we may have to cancel if [the patient] isn't feeling well that day. We'll try to give you as much notice as possible. Is that okay?"

12. Respect the limits of others.

"It was very hard when Grandma said she wanted to be alone for the holidays. Grandpa had died in May, and she was in the middle of chemotherapy. I hated the idea that she might be alone. I offered to pay for a plane ticket, to come down and get her, to take our family there. I'd do anything, but she refused.

"In the end a friend said, 'Let it go. She needs to do this her way. She has a lot of adjustments to make. As much as she might want to be around you, she needs to be alone, to be in her home, in her bed, among her friends and her belongings.'

"I stopped pushing her. Now I realize that my grandmother knew how to set limits. Later, she thanked me for respecting her wishes."

13. Enjoy the doing, not just the end result.

Enjoying the doing is especially vital during the holidays, when the sorrows of cancer patients and their families are magnified. Appreciate every small victory, every meaningful moment. You can be the person who helps them see how precious these times are.

14. Do something for someone else.

- Get some friends together, and go caroling at a local hospital, nursing home, or shelter. Bring cookies or homemade muffins for the people you entertain.
- Donate clothes, decorations, or blankets to a charity.
- Work the phones during a charity telethon.
- Help serve Thanksgiving dinner at a shelter.
- If the patient or caregiver is someone you work with, give a small tasteful gift. Hand-deliver it before the holiday. Enclose a personal note written on your own stationery.
- Choose an idea from Chapter 5, and give a gift to someone you care about.
- Include your child when you do things for others.

15. Give yourself a gift.

Use Chapter 5 to get ideas for a gift for yourself, or do one of the following:

- Take an evening to reread all of your old holiday cards.
- Spend the holiday with a glass of wine, a fire, and a good friend. Talk about past holidays and dreams for the future. Look at each other's family photo albums, scrapbooks, or high school yearbooks.
- Ask the baby-sitter to come two hours early. Take a relaxing bubble bath before you get ready, or use the time to get your hair styled or your nails manicured. Or have a quiet leisurely drink with your loved one before you go out.
- Keep the baby-sitter for an hour longer after you arrive home.

Use the time to have a cup of tea and talk about the evening with your loved one.

- On Valentine's Day buy yourself flowers, a piece of jewelry, a new golf club, or an hour with a masseuse or personal trainer.
- Spend an evening with your kids, and don't answer the phone.
- Make calls to your long-distance friends throughout the holidays. An hour on the phone with a long-lost friend can make you feel revived. Take pleasure in their excitement when they receive your unexpected call.
- Don't make resolutions for this New Year's. Instead, reevaluate where you are, and acknowledge how much you've accomplished.
- A month before a holiday, take ten minutes every day to write down three things you're thankful for.
- Cuddle up with a good book for an entire afternoon.

One of the most important things you can do during a holiday is to spend time with people you enjoy, who give you strength, who let you be yourself and help you create feelings of hope.

I know this isn't always possible. You don't always get to choose whom you spend time with. But your life is different now. Your basket is only so big—fill it with as many roses, as many precious moments as you can.

The holidays can be a time to reaffirm your love for those around you. Counting your blessings, sharing goodwill, and being good to yourself are all ways to celebrate these milestones in your life.

If you plan a holiday well, it can generate positive feelings that spill over into the days that precede and follow it.

Part of learning to survive this disease is discovering when to celebrate the victories you and your loved one have achieved. A holiday is a perfect time to celebrate those accomplishments. But don't let it be the only occasion. Every time you learn something, help someone, or show that you care is a day, a moment to celebrate. You have the power to create these celebrations, to make life precious.

Epilogue

Cancer care has come a long way since I began my work in the field. Had my mother had this disease in the seventies, would she now be playing golf with her father, another cancer survivor, matching him stroke-by-stroke? Would they be looking into the eyes of the generations following them—grandchildren and great-grandchildren? Our society has also made tremendous progress in the way we talk about cancer, and in the way we treat people who are coping with it. And yet we have such a long journey left to travel. Those phone calls—the ones in which a voice announces someone you love is ill—still happen millions of times each year. And they don't happen to someone out there—they happen to us. I know, because two weeks ago Anne called—Anne, who cherished the stamps a friend once gave her; Anne, who has volunteered her time since 1984 to help families living with this disease. And like a missile shot across the wire, Anne announced, "I have kidney disease." Anne, why Anne? My treasured Anne, one of the closest friends I've ever had. Anne who has read almost every page of this book, carefully editing every word, every sentence. And so for me, the journey will start again. I am sure I will say things to her that I will later wish I hadn't. I won't do everything right. But I have something now—a guide I never had before. It is the voices, the advice of those who have been on this journey, the voices in this book. As Anne laughs into the phone, holding the pictures I just sent her of Lexi, I realize even more than I ever had, how helpless we are against any illness, and how powerful. We can give so much. We can do so much.

And as this book is helping me now, not only with Anne, but with friends and patients with many different kinds of illnesses. I hope it will give you the same comfort, the same guide, the same blanket to hold on to, the same anchor in the sea. The guidelines offered here will touch every area of your life. Following them will make you more aware, more alive, and hopefully more appreciative of all that you do have. I hope you are good to yourself, and that you don't wait for holidays to celebrate how special you are, how incredible every precious moment is.

Resources
(in alphabetical order)

Aging with Dignity
(888) 5-WISHES
http://www.agingwithdignity.org
A nonprofit organization that advocates for the needs of elders and their caregivers, with a particular emphasis on improving care for those at the end of life. Provides a living will.

Air Care Alliance
(918) 745-0384
http://www.aircareall.org
Promotes, supports, and represents the public through communication and cooperation among organizations facilitating flights for health, compassion, and community service.

Alliance for Aging
(202) 293-2856
http://www.agingresearch.org
A nonprofit citizen advocacy organization dedicated to improving the health and independence of Americans as they age, through advances in medical research. Promotes research for quality of life.

American Association for Geriatric Psychiatry
(301) 654-7850
http://www.aagpgpa.org
Dedicated to promoting the mental health and well-being of older people, improving the care of those with late-life mental disorders, and referrals for geriatric psychiatrists.

American Association of Retired Persons
(800) 424-3410
http://www.aarp.org
Offers free informational pamphlets and a magazine.

American Brain Tumor Association
(800) 886-2282
http://www.abta.org
Provides publications, maintains support group listings, and gives referrals to treatment facilities.

American Cancer Society
(800) ACS-2347
http://www.cancer.org
Divisions offer current information on treatments, third-party assistance, local resources, volunteers, and support groups. Your local unit may be able to arrange for durable medical equipment and supplies at no cost to the patient.

American Chronic Pain Association
(916) 632-0922
http://www.theacpa.org
Support for persons dealing with chronic pain.

American Foundation for Urologic Disease
(800) 828-7866
http://www.afud.org.
Provides magazine, information, and support on prostate cancer, kidney and other urological diseases, and impotence.

American Geriatrics Society
(212) 308-1414
http://www.americangeriatrics.org
Information on aging.

American Institute for Cancer Research
(800) 843-8114
http://www.aicr.org
Provides publications and videos on nutrition.

American Kidney Fund
(800) 638-8299
http://www.akfinc.org
Helps dialysis patients with transportation and medication needs.

American Liver Foundation
(800) GO-LIVER
http://www.liverfoundation.org
Gives information and provides a help line.

American Lung Association
(800) LUNG-USA
http://www.lungusa.org
Offers smoking cessation groups and issues literature on lung disease.

American Nurses Association
(202) 651-7000
http://www.nursingworld.org
A full-service professional organization representing the nation's entire registered nurse population.

American Pain Society
(847) 375-4715
http://www.ampainsoc.org
Provides a directory of U.S. pain centers.

American Psychiatric Association
(888) 357-7924
http://www.psych.org
Health information for patients and physicians.

American Psychological Association
(202) 336-5500
http://www.apa.org
Resource center for psychological issues.

American Red Cross
(202) 737-8300
http://www.redcross.org
Provides community services, including nursing health programs.

American Self-Help Clearinghouse
http://www.mentalhelp.net/selfhelp
Lists self-help groups.

American Society for Clinical Hypnosis
(630) 980-4760
http://www.asch.net
Lists members in your area.

American Society of Clinical Oncology
(703) 299-0150
http://www.asco.org
Offers updated information on treatments and clinical findings.

Anderson Network
(800) 392-1611
http://www.mdanderson.org
Provides peer support through a telephone network and holds an annual conference.

**Asian & Pacific Islander
American Health Forum**
(415) 954-9988
http://www.apiahf.org
Dedicated to promoting policy, program, and research efforts for the improvement of health status of all Asian-American and Pacific Islander communities.

Association of Cancer Online Resources
http://www.acor.org
Cancer information system currently offers access to electronic mailing lists and a variety of web sites.

Association of Oncology Social Work
(847) 375-4721
http://www.aosw.org
Dedicated to increasing awareness about the social, emotional, educational, and spiritual needs of cancer patients.

Bloch Cancer Foundation, Inc.
(800) 433-0464
http://www.blochcancer.org
Provides resources, peer counseling, second opinions, and support groups.

Blood & Marrow Transplant Newsletter
(888) 597-7674
http://www.bmtinfonet.org
Publishes a newsletter, provides medical information, and offers patients and loved ones support.

Breast Cancer Hotline
(212) 382-2111
http://www.sharecancersupport.org
Provides support services for women, men, and children who have been affected by breast or ovarian cancer.

Cancer Care, Inc.
(800) 813-HOPE
http://www.cancercare.org
Social workers provide free one-to-one, group, and telephone counseling; online and free teleconferences; worksite programs; and referrals. Publishes brochures and a newsletter.

Cancer Club
(800) 586-9062
http://www.cancerclub.com
Offers humorous and helpful books, cassettes, and a newsletter.

Cancer Counseling, Inc.
(713) 520-9873
Free professional counseling and educational programs provided by psychologists, social workers, and psychiatrists.

Cancer Facts
http://www.cancerfacts.com
Provides personalized, interactive treatment information.

Cancer Hope Network
(877) HOPENET
http://www.cancerhopenetwork.org
Trained survivors offer counseling to those undergoing chemotherapy and radiation.

Cancer Information Service (CIS)
See **National Cancer Institute's Cancer Information Service.**

Cancer Legal Resource Center
(213) 736-1455
http://www.wlcdr.everybody.org/cancer.mason
Provides information and educational outreach on cancer-related legal issues to people with cancer, their families, friends, employers, and those who provide services to them.

Cancer Source
(978) 579-8226
http://www.cancersource.com
Contains general information about cancer and links to news articles.

Cancer Survivor's Network
http://www.cancersurvivorsnetwork.org
Covers coping with fear, financial planning, and long-term effects of treatment.

Cancervive
(310) 203-9232
http://www.cancervive.org
Helps cancer survivors face and overcome the challenges of "life after cancer."

Candlelighters Childhood Cancer Foundation
(800) 366-2223
http://www.candlelighters.org
Focuses on families of children with cancer and children who are long-term survivors.

CANSearch
http://www.cansearch.org/canserch/canserch.htm
Lists Internet resources.

CaP Cure
(800) 757-CURE
http://www.capcure.org
Prostate cancer research and information.

Caregivers, Inc.
(954) 893-0550
http://www.caregiver.com
Information on caregivers in the workforce.

CDC National AIDS Hotline
(800) 342-2437 (24 hours)
Hotline provides information, referral services, and publications about HIV and AIDS.

CenterWatch
(617) 856-5900
http://www.centerwatch.com
Lists clinical trials that are recruiting patients and gives background information on clinical research.

Children's Hospice International
(800) 242-4453
http://www.chionline.org
Provides resources and referrals to children with life-threatening conditions and their families.

Children's Oncology Camps of America
(803) 434-3503

Colon Cancer Alliance
(877) 422-2030
http://www.ccalliance.org
Provides patient support services and facilitates access to information.

Colorectal Cancer Awareness Month
(877) 422-2030
http://www.preventcancer.org
Offers a toll-free hotline, buddy program, educational materials, resources, and clinical trial information.

Colorectal Cancer Registry at Johns Hopkins
(888) 77-COLON
email:hccregistry@wpmail.onc.jhu.edu
Information on genetic screening and counseling.

Compassionate Friends
(630) 990-0010
Resource guide for grief.

Conversations!
(806) 355-2565
http://www.ovarian-news.org
Newsletter for families coping with ovarian cancer.

Cure for Lymphoma Foundation
(800) CFL-6848
http://www.cfl.org
Provides support and education to families touched by Hodgkin's disease and non-Hodgkin's Lymphoma.

Eldercare Locator Service
(800) 677-1116
http://www.aoa.dhhs.gov
Nationwide directory assistance service.

Family Caregiver Alliance
(415) 434-3388
http://www.caregiver.org
Clearinghouse for services related to brain impairments.

Food and Drug Administration
(888) 463-6332
http://www.fda.gov
Information on specific drugs.

Gilda's Club
(888) 445-3248
http://www.gildasclub.org
A free community support group that provides art activities, social events, and emotional support.

Gillette Women's Cancer Connection
(800) 688-9777
Lists support groups, resources, and provides brochures.

Grief, Mourning, and Depression
(800) 421-4211
NIMH Depression Awareness, Recognition and Treatment Program.

Griefnet
http://www.rivendell.org
Resource for coping with grief.

Gynecologic Cancer Foundation
(800) 444-4441
http://www.wcn.org/gcf
Provides newsletter, medical referrals, public education materials; involved in activities for Gynecological Awareness Month (September); and provides online risk assessment.

Health Insurance Association of America
(202) 824-1600
http://www.hiaa.org
Advocate for privately based health care.

Health Insurance & Financial Resources
(800) 932-0050
http://www.nvrnvr.com
Information on insurance policies.

Healthfinder
http:///www.healthfinder.gov
Medical dictionary and links to medical journals and health-related sites.

Hospice Foundation of America
(800) 854-3402
http://www.hospicefoundation.org
Assists those who cope either personally or professionally with terminal illness, death, and the process of grief. Information on how to select a home-care agency; lists hospices; answers questions on caregiving, living with grief; and provides a monthly newsletter.

Intercultural Council
(713) 798-4617
Works to eliminate unequal burden of cancer in racial and ethnic minorities.

International Association of Laryngectomees
(800) 227-2345

International Myeloma Foundation
(800) 452-CURE
http://www.myeloma.org
Publishes a newsletter and brochures; sponsors support groups and conferences; and provides web site links to clinical trials.

Intouch
(516) 777-3800
http://www.intouchlive.com
Magazine with articles about cancer prevention, social and emotional aspects of cancer, nutrition, clinical trials, and up-to-date treatments.

Joint Commission on Accreditation of Healthcare Organizations Public Information Coordinator Department of Corporate Relations
(630) 792-5000
http://www.jcaho.org
Accredits hospitals.

Kids Konnected
(800) 899-2866
http://www.kidskonnected.org
Serves children of parents with cancer; provides newsletters, referrals, and support.

Susan G. Komen Breast Cancer Foundation
(800) 462-9273
http://www.breastcancerinfo.com
Operates a breast cancer helpline and works to advance research, education, screening, and treatment of breast cancer.

Leukemia Society of America
(800) 955-4LSA (educational materials)
(212) 573-8484 (general information)
http://www.leukemia.org
Provides research, patient aid, brochures, referrals, and support groups.

Lighthouse International
(800) 829-0500
http://www.lighthouse.org
Resource for visually impaired.

Look Good...Feel Better
(800) 395-LOOK
Helps people improve their appearance during treatment.

Lymphoma Research Foundation of America, Inc.
(800) 500-9976
http://www.lymphoma.org
Provides "buddy" program, conference, and newsletter.

Make Today Count
(608) 263-8521
http://www.userpages.itis.com/lemoll/index/html
Provides emotional support to survivors and their families.

Managed Care Made Easy
http://www.peoplesmed.org
Complete guide on HMOs.

M. D. Anderson Cancer Center
http://www.mdanderson.org
Lists clinical trials.

Medscape
http://www.medscape.com
Interactive web site on clinical studies and medical articles.

National Alliance of Breast Cancer Organizations
(800) 719-9154
http://www.nabco.org
A clearinghouse for breast cancer information and assistance; provides a resource guide and a newsletter.

National Association of Social Workers
(800) 638-8799
http://www.naswdc.org
Works to enhance the professional growth and development of its members, to create and maintain professional standards, and to advance sound social policies.

National Bone Marrow Transplant Link
(800) Link-BMT
http://comnet.org/nbmtlink
Provides peer support and information.

National Brain Tumor Foundation
(800) 934-2873
http://www.braintumor.org
Provides support and education.

National Breast Cancer Coalition
(800) 622-2838
http://www.natlbcc.org
Advocacy organization that promotes active participation in making treatment decisions.

National Cancer Institute's Cancer Information Service
(800) 4-CANCER (CIS)
http://www.nci.nih.gov
*The nationwide telephone service and its web sites provide
free printed and web-based materials, referrals and information on treatment options, clinical trials, research and news.
Ask for "Taking Time; Facing Forward" and brochures on
medical aspects of cancer, such as coping with chemotherapy.*

National Cancer Survivors Day Foundation
(615) 794-3006
http://www.ncsdf.org
Organizes Survivors Day on the first Sunday in June.

National Childhood Cancer Foundation
(800) 458-6223
http://www.nccf.org
Newsletter provides up-to-date information on research.

National Children's Cancer Society
(800) 532-6459
http://www.children-cancer.com
*Programs for children in need of bone marrow transplant
services.*

National Coalition for Cancer Survivorship
(877) 622-7937
http://www.cansearch.org
*Specializes in work-related rights and insurance benefits; pro-
vides free educational materials, including audio programs for
developing practical skills for daily living.*

National Comprehensive Cancer Network
(888) 909-NCCN
http://www.nccn.org
Provides a referral service on informed decision-making.

National Family Caregivers Association
(800) 896-3650
http://www.nfcacares.org
Helps caregivers by providing research, education, support, and a resource guide. Distributes a newsletter with practical tips on caregiving.

National Hospice Organization
(800) 658-8898
http://www.nho.org
Provides educational publications and programs, and referrals to national and international hospices.

National Institute of Allergy and Infectious Diseases
http://www.niaid.nih.gov
Information on clinical trials and up-to-date news.

National Kidney Cancer Association
(800) 850-9132
http://www.nkca.org
A membership organization made up of patients, family members, physicians, researchers, and other health professionals.

National Library of Medicine
http://www.nlm.nih.gov
Information on clinical trials and abstracts from medical journals.

National Lymphedema Network
(800) 293-3362
http://www.lymphnet.org
Provides data bank, online education and referrals; publishes a newsletter; and acts as an advocate.

National Mental Health Association
(800) 433-5959
http://www.nmha.org
Resource for dealing with mental illness.

National Organization for Rare Disorders
(800) 999-6673
http://www.rarediseases.org
Organization that works toward the prevention, treatment, and cure of rare "orphan" diseases.

National Ovarian Cancer Coalition
(888) 682-7426
http://www.ovarian.org
Organization committed to improving the overall survival and quality of life from ovarian cancer.

Needy Meds
http://www.needymeds.com
Lists pharmaceutical manufacturers that help people who can't afford medication. Includes information on possible drug interactions.

ONCOLINK
http://www.oncolink.com
Information, resources, and book reviews for health care personnel, patients, and their loved ones.

Oncology.com
http://www.oncology.com
Up-to-date source of online cancer news and information for patients and health care professionals.

Oncology Nursing Society
(412) 921-7373
http://www.ons.org
National organization of more than 30,000 registered nurses and other health care professionals dedicated to excellence in patient care, teaching, research, administration, and education in the field of oncology.

Ovarian Cancer National Alliance
(202) 331-1332
http:///www.ovariancancer.org
Newsletter provides medical updates and information on clinical trials, and other aspects of ovarian cancer.

Partnership for Caring
(800) 989-WILL
http://www.partnershipforcaring.org
Provides individual counseling on living wills and medical powers of attorney. A living will is free if you fill it out online.

Patient Advocate Foundation
(800) 532-5274
http://www.patientadvocate.org
Seeks to safeguard patients through effective mediation assuring access to care, maintenance of employment and preservation of their financial stability.

Patient-Centered Guides
http://www.patientcenters.com
Comprehensive resources list of guides and books.

Problems with Family
(215) 945-6900
Services for children of aging parents.

Ronald McDonald House
(630) 623-7048
http://www.rmhc.com
Temporary housing for children with life-threatening illnesses and their families.

RxList
(510) 250-2500
http://www.rxlist.com
Provides prescription information.

Share
(212) 719-0364
http://www.sharecancersupport.org
Support services, including hotline and free groups, for women with ovarian or breast cancer.

Sisters Network, Inc.
(713) 781-0255
African-American cancer survivor's organization.

Skin Cancer Foundation
(800) 754-6490
http://www.skincancer.org
International organization that is concerned exclusively with cancer of the skin.

Stadtlanders Pharmacy and Ortho Biotech's National Oncology Resource Directory
(800) 238-7828
http://stadtlanders.com
A free brochure listing national resources and manufacturers of medications frequently prescribed for patients.

United Ostomy Association, Inc.
(800) 826-0826
http://www.uoa.org
Rehabilitation services for ostomates.

United States National Library of Medicine
(800) 338-7657
http://www.nlm.nih.gov

US TOO International, Inc.
(800) 808-7866
http://www.ustoo.com
Provides emotional support and educational materials.

Visiting Nurse Associations of America
(617) 523-4042
http://www.vnaa.org
Provides names of local visiting nurse associations and community-based home care services, including skilled nurses, therapists, and home health care aides.

WebMD
http://www.WebMD.com
Carries articles, columns, and chat transcripts by the author, and information and news on psychosocial and medical issues.

Well Spouse Foundation
(800) 838-0879
http://www.wellspouse.org
Provides support groups and newsletter.

World Health Organization Publications Center USA
http://www.who.int
Provides publications on pain management.

Y-ME
National Breast Cancer Organization
(800) 221-2141
http://www.yme.org
Provides telephone counseling and educational programs.

YWCA Encore Plus
(800) 953-7587
http://www.ywca.org
Discussion and exercise program for women who have had breast cancer surgery.

Index

Index

About the Author

Elise NeeDell Babcock is the founder of Cancer Counseling Inc., the first agency of its kind to provide free professional counseling to people coping with cancer during any stage of the disease. She and CCI were honored by M. D. Anderson Cancer Center as partners in the fight against cancer. She's written online articles for *USA Today* and CNN's WebMD. Elise was a radio co-host for *Talk America* for three years and she's lectured across the country at places such as Yale, Stanford, and Northwestern medical schools. She is on the board of *Intouch* magazine. She was the chairman of Operation Hope, a Houston forum on 9-11. She lives in Houston with her husband and daughter.

She can be contacted at:
Elise NeeDell Babcock
2001 Holcombe Suite 3702
Houston, Texas 77030
http://www.AskElise.com
eneedell@mail.org
(713) 796-9215